# Voices in the Band

A VOLUME IN THE SERIES

## THE CULTURE AND POLITICS OF HEALTH CARE WORK
Edited by Suzanne Gordon and Sioban Nelson

*A list of titles in this series is available at www.cornellpress.cornell.edu*

# Voices in the Band

A Doctor, Her Patients, and How
the Outlook on AIDS Care Changed
from Doomed to Hopeful

## Susan C. Ball

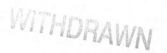

ILR Press
an imprint of
Cornell University Press
Ithaca and London

First published 2015 by Cornell University Press

Printed in the United States of America

Library of Congress Cataloging-in-Publication Data

Ball, Susan C., 1957– author.
    Voices in the band : a doctor, her patients, and how the outlook on AIDS care changed from doomed to hopeful / Susan C. Ball.
        pages cm — (The culture and politics of health care work)
    Includes bibliographical references and index.
    ISBN 978-0-8014-5362-5 (cloth : alk. paper)
    1. AIDS (Disease)—New York (State)—New York—History.
2. AIDS (Disease)—Patients—New York (State)—New York. I. Title.
II. Series: Culture and politics of health care work.
    RA643.84.N7B35    2015
    362.19697'920097471—dc23          2014034038

Cornell University Press strives to use environmentally responsible suppliers and materials to the fullest extent possible in the publishing of its books. Such materials include vegetable-based, low-VOC inks and acid-free papers that are recycled, totally chlorine-free, or partly composed of nonwood fibers. For further information, visit our website at www.cornellpress.cornell.edu.

Cloth printing          10 9 8 7 6 5 4 3 2 1

For Shari, Jules, and Paris

# Contents

Acknowledgments                                                ix

Author's Note                                                  xi

Introduction                                                    1

1. **1992**: Beginning                                         4

2. **1992**: So Much to Learn                                 18

3. **1992**: No Easy Answers and Little to Offer             33

4. **1994**: Too Many Drugs, No Medication                   47

5. **1994**: Being Mindful of the Subtext                    61

6. **1994**: Weekend on Call                                 75

7. **1994**: Christmas                                        88

8. **1995**: Another Support Group                          100

9. **1995**: Mothers and Children                           113

10. **1995**: Decisions and Revisions                       125

11. **1995**: Colleagues and Families                       138

12. **1995**: So Many Stories and Some New Faces            151

13. **1996**: Some Hope in the Despair            166

14. **1996**: Hit Early, Hit Hard                 181

15. **1997**: Amazing Changes                     195

16. **1999**: Despite Our Best Intentions         208

17. **1999**: Coping with a Different Paradigm    221

18. **2000**: Going Home                          234

Epilogue                                          248

# Acknowledgments

I could say that I began writing this book when I started my job at the Center for Special Studies—or maybe even before that, when I was writing about some of the patients I cared for while I was a resident or a medical student. I began consciously writing a book about ten years ago with the encouragement of my boss, Jon Jacobs. I wrote on and off, plugging away at times and leaving it in a drawer at others. Ultimately it was my partner, Shari, who, on seeing the advertisement for the Narrative Medicine Program at Columbia University in the *New Yorker* magazine, excitedly showed it to me and said, "You should do this, Suze; then you can finish your book." And she was right.

I had great teachers at the Narrative Medicine Program. Maura Siegel, Craig Irvine, Sayantani Das Gupta, Nellie Herman, Marsha Hurst, and Pat Stanley offered inspiration in this important field, and I thank them all. Rita Charon shepherded the program into being, and her support for the book has been enthusiastic and unflagging. I am indebted to her as an advisor, a colleague, and a friend. My superb writing teacher, Lynne Sharon Schwartz, spent countless hours reading and rereading, coaxing stronger sentences and intelligible phrasing from my passive-voice-prone pen. I am so grateful for her patient, meticulous help.

I hope it is clear in the story how much I admire Jon Jacobs. Jon has stood by me as a friend and mentor for more than twenty years. From the very start he has kept our focus on one essential ideal: to do what is best for the patient.

I hope this book conveys how we tried, always, to do that. Sam Merrick has also been a tremendous colleague, a dedicated, smart, compassionate physician with whom it has been a real honor to practice medicine. Jon's and Sam's support have been invaluable. All my colleagues at CSS have contributed to this book over the years, in ways great and small. I have been very fortunate to work among such an elite and committed group of professionals.

I cannot overstate my gratitude to my family. Writing a book while working as a full-time clinician meant a lot of early mornings or late nights alone with the computer with the door closed. My sons, Jules and Paris, got older; my partner did a lot of needlepoint and ordered take-out more than she would have liked. Through it all, Shari's unstinting belief in me, her patience, encouragement, and endless efforts to read and critique were phenomenal and wonderful, and I cannot possibly thank her enough.

Jamie Zimmerman and her daughters, Zoe and Charlotte, should not go unmentioned. Even when I couldn't find anything good to report they urged me to keep going, and they believed in me. I also thank Jim, Margo, Sarah, ML, Ray, and Joni for their support. Emily Wheeler provided wise comments and advice, and our long friendship helped me enormously. My dear friend Elizabeth Kelly continues to be a source of inspiration with her dedication and commitment to her important, sometimes lonely work in Cincinnati.

I owe a debt to Randy Shilts's, *"And the Band Played On,"* a book of heartbreaking integrity, which opened so many eyes and from whose title mine has borrowed.

I'd like to thank my editors and the talented, wonderful people at Cornell University Press. They have been welcoming and kind, thoughtful and perceptive. I enormously appreciate their belief in me and their support for the book.

Last I thank the hundreds of patients who contributed to the writing of this book. I hope some day we will cure AIDS and the time described in these pages will be just a shiver in history. But the patients will always be remembered.

# Author's Note

This is a work of narrative nonfiction. The events and people are real and the conversations took place. Memory, however, is the medium through which all of these words passed on their way to the written page. There are events, and then there is our memory of those events, and thereafter there is the memory of the memory. As a result, it's unlikely that any conversation or comment is documented verbatim and I do not pretend otherwise. I tried hard to be true to my sense of the moment, my appreciation for others' thoughts and feelings, and my respect for the individuals around me.

All the patients in these pages exist, but their names have been changed and identifiers are scrambled. People who know the clinic or have worked there will no doubt recognize some characters, but I tried to make each patient a composite of patients. I asked for and obtained permission from patients to include aspects of their stories in this book.

The names of all of my colleagues except my own and that of Dr. Jon Jacobs have been changed.

I should also say that there is a great deal that this book does not cover. Writing about ten years of HIV involved omitting much more than including. For example, I mention but in no way do justice to the activism of that period of time, and the dramatic influence of that activism on drug development and government involvement. I do not discuss the global impact of this epidemic, or how it continues to rage and decimate families and communities around the world, particularly in sub-Saharan Africa. I don't discuss Ronald Reagan and the sad cost of his bigotry, or the heroism of Larry Kramer, whom many reviled but who spoke the truth very early on. Or the amazing story of Ryan White, whose legacy continues to keep thousands of HIV-infected patients safe, so long after the young man died. This book is the story of one place and one time and the people who came and went in those moments.

# Voices in the Band

What is the course of the life
Of mortal men on the earth?—
Most men eddy about
Here and there—eat and drink,
Chatter and love and hate,
Gather and squander, are raised
Aloft, are hurl'd in the dust,
Striving blindly, achieving
Nothing; and, then they die—
Perish; and no one asks
Who or what they have been,
More than he asks what waves
In the moonlit solitudes mild
Of the midmost Ocean, have swell'd,
Foam'd for a moment, and gone.

MATTHEW ARNOLD, "RUGBY CHAPEL," ST. 6 (1867)

# Introduction

I am an AIDS doctor. I originally did my residency training in internal medicine, and in 1992 I started working for Dr. Jon Jacobs at the Center for Special Studies, the AIDS care center in New York City. At that time the idea of an HIV specialist was in its infancy. While we knew what caused AIDS, how it spread, and how to avoid getting it, we didn't know how to treat it or how to prevent our patients' seemingly inevitable progression toward death. The stigma that surrounded AIDS patients from the very beginning of the epidemic in the early 1980s continued to be harsh and isolating: mention AIDS and people imagined promiscuous homosexuals and heroin addicts, all of them skinny and covered with purple spots. They remembered those early photos of diaper-clad, emaciated men with scraggly beards looking fearfully into the face of the priest or nun leaning over their hospital bed. People looked askance at me: What was it like to work in that kind of environment with those kinds of people?

My patients are "those kinds of people." They are an array and a combination of brave, depraved, strong, entitled, admirable, self-centered, amazing, strange, funny, daring, gifted, exasperating, wonderful, and sad. And more. At my clinic most of the patients are indigent and few have had an education beyond high school, if that. Many are gay men and many of the patients use or have used drugs. They all have HIV, and in the early days far too many of them died. Every day they brought us the stories of their lives. We listened to them and we took care of them as best we could. My patients have the kinds of voices that are rarely heard, coming as they do from a hip-wiggling drag queen or a drug-using Hispanic man who lives in a shelter, or from a welfare-dependent single mother of four who lives in her subsidized two-bedroom sixth-floor walk-up out in a remote part of the city that I will likely never see. My colleagues and I heard the stories; and in caring for our patients we created more stories, with all the small victories, the horrible deaths, the humor, and the sadness. We worked hard to be good doctors and our patients helped us become better ones as we took our tumultuous journey together.

I wanted to write a book about my patients and my colleagues and how we made it through the roller-coaster last decade of the twentieth century, how we moved from helplessly watching our patients die to being able to offer them a treatment course and a fairly normal life expectancy. In that time we saw some patients literally return from death's door. This kind of dramatic success has not been seen in any other field of medicine, except perhaps following the introduction of penicillin many years ago. I wanted to try to answer the question "What was it like?" What was it like to care for patients with AIDS, a disease that didn't even exist when I was in college? How did we deal with dying patients for whom we had a diagnosis but no treatment? How did we care for patients that many in society rejected, patients that many even within the field of medicine rejected? What happened in those years, when the prognosis for a patient with HIV went from nearly hopeless to very hopeful?

The advances of medicine in the last twenty years or so have introduced ever more sophisticated technology, persistent clamoring for cost control, streamlined algorithms for patient care, and a lopsided two-tiered system divided between the rich and the poor. My experiences caring for patients with HIV brought me up against some of the best and worst aspects of medicine as I tried to care for patients who often were born into bad circumstances or made bad choices or were burdened with mental illness, domestic violence, or lack of family or education.

This is a book about HIV and AIDS and an important period in the history of the epidemic, but there is more to it, as I found in its writing. The care and treatment of patients with AIDS has changed, but the disease itself has not, nor have those who suffer from it, though they have shifted further out on the margins of our society. I want to tell people about these patients and how I cared for some of them during that time at our large academic medical center in New York City. Those years and experiences changed me as well, as I made the transition from trying to help patients as they died to trying to help them live long, healthy lives.

My colleagues and I struggled to care for the poorest of the poor and the sickest of the sick, and this book follows the stories of several of those patients. But as the smothering blanket of mortal illness gradually lifted from our patients, we could see a deeper story emerging. We could recognize the tremendous value of our multidisciplinary approach and how each and every patient helped us along the way. We learned as doctors, as a team, and as people; each of us vulnerable, each of us trying to do the best we could.

In the end, it is the patients who are at the heart of this story.

I am an AIDS doctor. For more than twenty years I have taken care of many patients and I am happy to say that Stewart and Olive are doing well.

I took care of Etta. And I wish that she had taken her medication.

# Chapter One

# 1992 Beginning

After all of these years, I still remember that egg, a half-eaten hard-boiled egg held delicately in his dark, slender fingers. The egg had a bite taken out of it and he was looking at the egg with a perplexed expression, as if he wasn't quite sure what he held. The whites of his large eyes shone brightly. His eyelashes were long and dusty looking. I stood next to his bed and leaned in a bit to look at him with my face on his level. He smiled at me, showing partially eroded gums and a lot of egg in and around his teeth. I wanted him to put the egg down. I didn't want to see him take another bite of it. Please, I found myself thinking, please don't take another bite.

The several vases in Mac's hospital room held flowers that were long dead. Milk and juice cartons cluttered every surface. Crumbs and items from his breakfast tray, including what appeared to be most of the shell and peelings from the egg, covered the pale blue blanket on his bed. A navy baseball cap with a stiff brim sat sideways on his head. One of Mac's friends had decorated the hat with plastic eyes and pink glitter.

I smiled back at him and said, "Hello, Mac, how are you today?"

Mac blinked slowly and I tried to avoid looking at those teeth. His long lashes rested on his cheeks. "Hello, doc."

"Can I sit down?"

He nodded yes and I sat at the end of his bed. I could see where his very skinny legs raised the blankets and I made sure not to sit on them. "How is your breakfast going there?"

"Oh, it's all right, I guess."

I watched as he slowly put his egg down on the tray. I was thinking, leave-it-there-leave-it-there-leave-it-there. He delicately picked up an empty packet of sugar and turned it over.

"How is your appetite?"

"All right, I guess."

We were silent for a minute or so. Mac tried to pour the empty packet of sugar into what I was certain was a cold cup of coffee. Several open packets of sugar had already been emptied onto the tray.

"Are you getting out of bed?"

He smiled again and watched the sugar packet in his fingers. "Not today. Not yet."

Silence. Mac moved slowly. It was like watching a movie frame by frame. I heard a nurse calling to someone out in the hallway. Mac turned the sugar packet again in his fingers. I sat up straighter to ease my back but I didn't look away from Mac's face. I wanted him to see that I was focused only on him.

"Mac, if the nurses come and help you, will you get out of bed and sit in a chair today?"

"I might."

"Do you want to?"

He turned the sugar packet a couple of times without looking up.

"I might."

I felt a flicker of worry. The day, my work, the rounds, the notes and meetings and phone calls, it all waited out there for me, tapping its foot. I didn't want to feel impatient and I didn't want Mac to feel that I was impatient. But we needed to move forward. I needed Mac to answer my questions and I needed to have him hear the words; even when I knew that he could no longer organize his thoughts the way he once had, the way a healthy man at his age should.

"Mac, I spoke to your sister Laverne and also to Briana. You remember Briana, your social worker? She spoke to Laverne as well. We were talking about whether you can go home or not."

Mac continued to work silently at the empty sugar packet in his slender fingers.

"Mac, Laverne cannot care for you at her house. You know that, right?"

"I don't want to go to her house."

"Well, Mac, we can't let you go back to your house. We can't let you go back there to live."

Mac didn't say anything. I waited.

Finally, after putting down the empty sugar packet he said, "I would like to go back there, to my own house."

I didn't answer him right away. "I know," I said, nodding. "I know that's what you want. I know that's where you'd like to be. But, Mac, for now you're just not strong enough to go there. We can't let you go there on your own. And Laverne can't look after you enough." I put my hand on the blanket and felt his skinny leg.

"You have been talking about me," he said.

"Yes, I know, we have been." I nodded again as I spoke.

He was looking at his tray and his hand absently strayed up to brush away a piece of egg that clung to his lip. He didn't look up.

I felt suddenly tired. It seemed clear that I was talking for me and that Mac was lost. He didn't understand. He was being polite and saying words that would fit into the mold of our conversation. I looked at him and felt this little tug somewhere, maybe in my shoulder, maybe in my hand, to reach out to this man who no longer commanded himself, who couldn't say anything more complicated or articulate than that he wanted to go home. Still, I had to keep going. "We talked together, Briana and I, and we talked to Laverne. And now I am talking to you to see how you are."

He swiped again at the bit of egg on his lip. "I want to go home."

"I know."

He picked up a spoon and held it carefully.

"We just—we just can't let you go back to your house, Mac. You wouldn't be safe there on your own. You can't get out of bed. You need a lot of care."

"Yeah." Mac put his spoon into the Styrofoam coffee cup and started stirring. He did seem to be listening. He blinked a few times. His eyelashes were so long.

I kept going, wanting to be done. "Mac, our thought is—and what we are going to try to do is—to get you to a place where you can get some good nursing care. I hope that if you rest a bit and get a little of your strength back, then maybe, well, let's just see if you can get a little stronger."

He looked up at me and blinked. He gave me a slow smile that lit up his face entirely, like someone cranking up the dimmer switch in a previously shadow-filled room. Despite the lingering presence of some egg, I could see there the sweet sexiness and charm that he surely once flaunted. I looked at that smile and sensed myself holding my breath. I smiled back at him.

Mac was thirty-three years old. Less than three months ago he had been working as a fashion assistant somewhere near Thirty-fourth Street and in the evenings whooping it up downtown with a pile of friends. I had just told this thirty-three-year-old man that he needed to go to a nursing home. He smiled at me and as I smiled back I thought, oh damn, this really stinks.

"Mac," I said, "we're going to talk some more about this. Have a little more breakfast, OK? I'll see you later." I saw that he'd looked back down at his tray and his fingers strayed toward the egg as I left his room. I shook my head and looked at the polished gray linoleum floor. What was happening? How had this happened?

But there it was: 1992 at one of the most prestigious medical centers in the city of New York, even in the whole country. The AIDS epidemic was roaring through the big cities in the Northeast, clustering in Miami and Atlanta, and ravaging the gay populations of San Francisco and Los Angeles. I was seeing Mac on rounds on one of the first days at my job as an attending physician on the HIV service at one of the New York–very–big–deal hospitals, an Ivy League–incredibly–smart medical center. I had joined the staff of the Center for Special Studies, the young HIV/AIDS clinic, and I'd assumed the care of 130 patients, ten of whom were in the hospital. There were three full-time and three part-time physicians caring for five hundred HIV-infected patients at our clinic. No one wanted to come to a clinic with HIV or AIDS in its name. No one wanted to be associated with such an awful diagnosis; the Center was thus named to protect our patients. People who had tested positive for the virus came to our clinic that had started as a one-room outpatient site three years prior. The Center itself had opened in 1991 after a beautiful renovation of the entire top floor of the hospital. We shared the space with the group doing clinical research on some of the various HIV medications that were in development.

Our inpatient floor operated twelve floors below the clinic. Before seeing Mac in his hospital room, I had seen five others so far that day. I'd seen Nilson of the perpetual scowl and John of the wondrously immaculate manicure. Both of them had *Pneumocystis* pneumonia. I'd seen Yolanda with raging herpes simplex and Hank who, while nearly falling asleep, was asking me for more morphine. Admitted for multiple complaints, Olive was undergoing tests but didn't seem to have anything wrong at all.

All ten of my patients in the hospital had AIDS, and half of them were dying. In 1992 no one knew how to treat patients with AIDS. We'd made some progress recognizing and treating some of the opportunistic infec-tions that we saw—infections that take advantage of a weakened immune system—but often the patients came into our offices and emergency rooms with problems we'd never encountered and had no idea how to treat: weird rashes or inexplicable shortness of breath; sudden inability to walk or rapid worsening of eyesight. Maybe some of this would become routine; we didn't know. The epidemic was moving into its second decade and still our emergency rooms and hospitals held too many dying patients for whom we had no diagnosis other than AIDS.

Mac's soft, doe-like gaze stayed with me as I sat down at the nursing station. The guy could barely feed himself. His thoughts and words seemed like those of a man in his nineties, not his thirties. He couldn't get out of bed but he wanted to be in his own apartment. His thoughts were slow and disorganized, but essentially he wanted what it is so natural to want. Especially in times of stress or fear or anxiety, we all want a little corner of some place to have as our own, a quiet haven or sanctuary. No different from anyone else, Mac wanted his familiar walls around him, his familiar window and curtains and cat lying on the Oriental rug. But he couldn't get up on his own. He couldn't get himself a glass of water or take a shower. He couldn't eat and he couldn't appreciate how totally helpless he was. So I talked to him about nursing homes. I talked to him about getting stronger. It felt dishonest to me. I smiled and looked into his face and did not tell him that it was completely unlikely to think that he would ever go home. I did not tell him that we had nothing further to offer him here at our big, important hospital.

His mental deterioration made him docile and quiet. He didn't rage or scream. Perhaps this made the acceptance easier in some ways, for his family and for him. But the horror of his progressive decline was hard to take in. His illness had forced changes in his life that none of us would have imagined. He wore diapers. When the nurses helped him up to sit next to the bed he needed to have a sheet wrapped around him and tied to the back of the chair so that he would not fall out of it. He could no longer brush his teeth. He didn't have pain. He could eat a little, when he was up to it, but a meal seemed to take hours and he left much more on the tray or the bed than he actually ingested. He had AIDS, that's all we knew; no other specific infection or cancer or stroke or anything that we could pin our puffed-up medical opinions on. A scan of his head showed only a vast shrinking of the undulating matter of his brain, with big, dark blackness where there should have been functioning white matter. And for this we knew of no treatment. So we watched and the nurses watched and those who loved him watched helplessly as his condition worsened and the man they knew faded away.

At the nurses' station my colleague Stan sat writing his progress notes. One of the people on his inpatient list was a twenty-six-year-old gay man named Edward, whose parents had come this morning from Florida because he was dying. His partner had died a year ago and now he was on the same path. I'd seen the parents earlier in the hall and they both looked fragile and dazed. Such a nice guy; quiet, friendly, unassuming, and in the last four months Edward had lost more and more weight and never received a diagnosis beyond advanced immune suppression. The nurses really liked him and could not have been more kind to the parents. Stan struggled with Edward's approaching death as well. There were scans and blood cultures and specialist consultations, but Edward had AIDS and that was all we really could say.

"How's Edward?" I asked Stan as I sat down next to him and pulled Mac's chart from the rack.

"Dying. Morphine drip." Stan didn't look up from writing in the chart. There were three other charts in a pile next to him.

"How are his parents doing?"

"Mother's a wreck, father doesn't talk." He lifted his head a bit and wiggled his pen in his fingers, still looking at the chart where he'd been writing. "They are so sweet, so . . . ," he paused, "so *nice*. They asked me if he could get some ice cream with his lunch. The guy hasn't eaten in probably five weeks. I said, sure, of course he can have ice cream." He wasn't looking at me as he spoke. He shook his head. He gave what I'd call a half laugh. The half laugh over something so terrible it's come around to being funny. But it's not funny.

"How long has he been on the morphine drip?"

"Just since last night. But I don't think he's going to need it for very long."

"Has he spoken?"

"Nah," Stan said, now looking at me. "He can't really talk at this point, he barely opens his eyes."

"Oh brother."

"Yeah." He looked back down at his chart and started writing.

I sat next to Stan and looked at the chart in my hands. It had Mac's identification label stuck on the spine. A maroon plastic chart with all the data of a man's illness inside.

Suddenly there was a huge crash out in the hallway and the sound of breaking glass; a man yelling and a woman calling loudly for help. Everyone around me jumped up and looked toward the hallway. It seemed that all the people started yelling at once. The clerk grabbed the phone and, dialing furiously, called, "Where's security? Where is security?"

Stan quickly moved into the hall and shouted, "Dennis, get back in your room!" As I followed Stan to the hall I heard him say, "Broke the fucking window." He sounded surprised and he walked quickly toward the crash.

One of the nurses rushed toward us from down the hall and breathlessly said to the clerk, "Call security, and call Dr. Berry, stat. That Dennis, that guy, Jesus, he scared me. He threw his chair into the window. There's all glass in the hall. Damn that guy, he is like some kind of wild man. Judy, do you have any Haldol in your drawer?" She was breathing hard and put her hand on her chest over her blue scrub shirt. Her dark red hair had been pinned up and now fell in locks around her face.

Down the hall, the guy, Dennis, stood talking to Stan, who was at least a foot taller. Dennis's wrists trailed the long gauze restraints that had previously tied him to his bed. His hair and beard needed a trim. He wore two hospital gowns, one of them on backwards, and his feet were bare.

"My fucking lunch!" He suddenly yelled up into Stan's face.

"OK, Dennis, OK, your lunch is coming," Stan said in a cajoling, friendly voice. "Dennis, just get back in your room now. Dennis, come on, buddy, there's glass all over the floor." He gently put his hand on the patient's shoulder and walked him back into his room. Stan looked down the hall and saw me and raised his eyebrows. He gave an impressed nod of his head: the window really was broken.

I saw the cart with the lunch trays parked outside another patient's room three doors away. Instead of waiting for his lunch to be delivered, Dennis had thrown his chair through the window of the door to his room. It's always possible that they'd skipped him and not brought him lunch. Maybe he had a test scheduled and they hadn't brought him breakfast, either. Maybe, maybe. I imagined Dennis in a line at the Social Security office or at the office for Medicaid benefits. I remembered the time years ago when I went to the Social Security office myself because they'd confused my number with someone else's. I stood in line for over two hours to get to the woman who finally helped me. How would Dennis do in a long, snaking line like that, seeing the people behind the glass, the ones who were supposed to be helping, as they talked and laughed among themselves and seemed to be doing any number of random things: copying papers, talking on the phone, writing on a pad of paper, and basically ignoring the line on the other side of the glass? I'd been grumpy and impatient after two hours and I now shook my head, smiling to myself, thinking about a guy like Dennis waiting in that line. I thought of flying chairs and broken glass. At the Social Security office all the chairs were fastened to the floor and the glass divider between the office workers and those in line was about a foot thick. Now I knew why.

I heard Dr. Berry's name paged stat overhead. A nurse ran by holding a small bottle of something and a syringe. Two heavy security guards came hustling past, hurriedly putting on bright yellow gloves. AIDS patients freaked people out. The hospital security guards always wore yellow rubber gloves when they came to our floor. Annoying, ridiculous rubber gloves. The men looked like they were about to do the dishes. They stepped gingerly over the glass outside Dennis's door and went into his room.

I returned to the nurses' station and picked up Mac's chart. Soon Stan joined me, sitting down heavily in his chair. He was chuckling, shaking his head. "Can you imagine doing *that* for the food *here*?"

I laughed and asked him, "No one's hurt?"

"Jane's a little freaked. She thought he was going to throw the chair at *her*."

"I thought that glass was, like, bulletproof."

"It has that chicken wire in it but it sure is smashed. He got a little cut on his foot."

"What did they give him?"

"Vitamin H." Stan shook his head again. "Nothing like a little Haldol before lunch." He picked up his pen and continued writing his note.

Dennis had AIDS, too. Dennis and Mac and Edward, all with AIDS. I looked at the patient list I'd written on a half piece of progress note paper. My inpatients all had AIDS; that is, their HIV infection had progressed and their immune systems were compromised. People used the two terms as if they were synonymous: AIDS and HIV. But not every patient infected with HIV had a diagnosis of AIDS. HIV meant infection with the virus but AIDS meant the virus had beaten down the immune system, rendered one vulnerable to infections and cancers that the body can usually fight off.

As I looked at my list of ten patients I felt an ominous creeping sensation come over me. These names represented people in my care now. Were they all going to die? Was everyone on this list a living dead person? I shook my head, literally shook that thought right out. I could not think about my patients that way. I thought again about Mac and his beautiful smile and the egg all mushed in his teeth. I thought about Dennis barefoot in the hall with broken glass on the floor around him. No, these were very much living characters. I pictured their faces one by one. Edward, too, though dying, remained very much alive for those who loved him, including his parents and the nurses.

We had so much to learn about AIDS, a disease that we knew best as frightening and unpredictable. The epidemic started quietly in the United States with clusters of unusual illnesses among gay men. I was a first-year medical student in 1982 when I heard the expression gay-related immune deficiency (GRID). No one knew what caused it, no one could predict which gay man would get it. Within two years GRID had evolved into acquired immune deficiency syndrome (AIDS), and those at risk included gay men, injection drug users, hemophiliacs, and Haitians. Soon a few women and some children joined the lists of those diagnosed with the illness. By 1985 the human immunodeficiency virus (HIV) had been identified as the causative agent. It became clear that AIDS arose from a viral infection that could be transmitted through sex, blood, shared needles, and from a pregnant mother to her unborn child. Pooled blood products had caused nearly every hemophiliac in the country to be infected with HIV prior to screening of the blood supply. Discovery of the virus led to the development of a straightforward blood test to determine whether an individual was infected with the virus through detection of an antibody, a protein made by the immune system. Screening of blood donors became mandatory in 1985, making transfusion-related transmission of HIV highly unlikely.

When I began working at the Center for Special Studies in 1992, my patients were fairly evenly divided among gay men, men who were current or former intravenous drug users, and women. About half of the women had acquired the infection from their sexual partners. The other half had been infected through intravenous drug use. Because many of our patients were indigent and few had jobs, government assistance paid for the medical care of most people being treated at CSS. So far I had met only one patient educated beyond high school.

Stan, our colleague Maggie, and I made up the full-time medical staff responsible for the majority of the five hundred HIV-positive patients enrolled in our clinic. Stan was easygoing and confident with his patients, in contrast to Maggie, who tended to be stressed out and anxious. Both of them had begun working at CSS a year before I got there, having just completed their residency training at the medical center. Maggie took me around on my first day and reviewed the patient list with me. She had nicknames for most of the patients or endearing comments to make about them, saying things like, he's a sweetie, I love her, he's an angel, he's such a peach, and so on. She expressed great worry and concern about several of the patients and she got teary-eyed telling me about them. She brushed the tears away, saying she'd not had a good night's sleep. I was struck by her sincerity but also by the intimate way in which she referred to her patients. I wondered if she could be effective if she was so emotionally involved. Having worked in a general medicine clinic for four years before coming to join Maggie and Stan, I had some experience and a sense of how I interacted with patients. These first days on the job introduced me to what my two colleagues had already been doing for a year, caring for patients with HIV and AIDS. It felt like I was hopping onto a fast train going off into a dark land, headlight slicing through the unknowable night.

With Dennis settled down, Stan finished his notes and headed back to the clinic. It was nearly two o'clock and time to go to support group. I put Mac's chart back on the rack and walked down the hall to take the elevator to the twenty-fourth floor. When I got to the conference room, people were already sitting in most of the big leather chairs around the table. I recognized many of the people and remembered most of their names. A small, unfamiliar woman with a lot of curly dark hair sat at one end, and she smiled at me as I sat down. Dr. Berry and Stan talked quietly together and I heard Stan say something about the fucking lunch that made Dr. Berry laugh. A few people, including Dr. Jacobs, came in behind me and chose to sit in the chairs that stood along the wall. The entire twenty-fourth floor had originally been the home of the hospital squash courts, and all of the rooms in our clinic have very high ceilings. In 1989 Dr. Jacobs had somehow persuaded the hospital to give up squash and take care of patients with HIV instead, a concept that now sounds amazing. I'm still not sure how he did it.

The woman with the dark curly hair looked at the clock, and then she looked at Dr. Jacobs. The room got quiet and Dr. Jacobs spoke up: "I'm glad everyone is here. This, as you know, is our support group. We haven't met in a while; maybe some of us are recovering from our last support group." There was some laughter and rolling of eyes. "We're happy to have a new support group leader with us today. This is Janice who is highly recommended. Let me just add that we will be meeting here at this time every other week, and again, all the care providers are invited and encouraged to be here." With that everyone looked at Janice, the woman with the curly hair, who said hello and looked around the room.

Janice gave a brief summary of her background and noted that she had led a couple of other support groups, including a group for HIV-positive men that met downtown. She had not facilitated a group of care providers such as ourselves but hoped we would all benefit from the time spent in that room.

It got very, very quiet.

No one spoke. Most people looked at the table in front of them. Occasionally someone would look up and meet the eyes of the person across the table. There were small smiles and then the eyes would go back to the tabletop. Here we are, I thought. All of us are here because we're taking care of patients with HIV. All the people in this room have chosen this work. I thought of Edward downstairs with his parents sitting there at his bedside. Waiting. I glanced at Stan. He'd told me yesterday that in the past year, thirty of his patients had died. Thirty! I thought of my patient John, who lay in a bed downstairs with his second case of *Pneumocystis* pneumonia and a collapsed lung. He still required oxygen but was recovering, it appeared. He'd seemed happy to meet me as his new doctor and had told me about his life. He loved his job as a stylist in a hair salon. He waved his hands around as he spoke and I watched them, entranced by his expressive gestures and perfectly polished fingernails. If he hadn't been wearing an oxygen mask he would not have looked sick. But he'd been admitted to the intensive care unit and only three days ago had been taken off a respirator and moved to the regular inpatient floor. Was John going to die very soon? He had only four CD4 cells. A healthy HIV-negative person usually has over five hundred of these cells—also called T cells. Without T cells John's immune system could no longer function adequately against certain kinds of infections.

I thought of Mrs. Perlucci, a woman I had taken care of last year before I came to work at CSS. Mrs. Perlucci died of pancreatic cancer after a brief but dramatic illness. In several short weeks I watched as she changed from an elegant elderly woman to an emaciated, yellow, wincing vision of death. It had been hard to be her doctor; so little to offer, so little difference to make. Did Stan watch that happen thirty times last year? Stan with his kind eyes and reassuring smile. Did he hold their hands and hug their parents? What about the social workers here in the room, or the nurses? Those thirty patients had been under their care as well. What do you say about how it feels? I found myself wondering, could I go through that? I'd chosen to be here. I wanted to work with these patients. I remember clearly that first support group and the almost overwhelming grief and loss that I sensed in the hearts of those around the table.

I wondered whether John's parents were alive and whether they knew that their son had AIDS. Edward's parents were with Edward. Would John's parents come to the bedside of this soft-spoken, handsome man and touch one of those beautifully manicured hands of his? I pictured an older woman washing her dinner dishes at a sink by a window. Turning to answer the telephone, she wipes her hands on her apron. I picture her sitting down with an anguished cry when she hears the news. I know this vision is out of a movie. Stan, Dr. Jacobs, the others around the room, they have been witnesses to indescribable sadness. The silence in the conference room seemed both deafening and endless. No one spoke, no one moved. Janice sat quietly with her hands folded on the table in front of her. She looked at us.

I found myself holding back tears. Should I talk about being afraid of all my patients dying? Should I mention that I felt unnerved by the degree of illness in my patients, all so sick and so young? All the people in the room, my colleagues, were like heroes to me, coming to work every day to care for dying patients that others shunned. I worried that I couldn't be as strong as they all seemed to be. I'd seen them chatting in the halls and joking in meetings. But no one underestimated the seriousness of the work. In that reverberating silence I heard everyone struggling to contain their own sorrow. Did my thoughts have any importance in the midst of all the despair and death that our patients were dealing with? Here we were in support group. I was the new kid; was I supposed to talk?

At the thought of opening my mouth to speak, my eyes filled with tears. I struggled to contain my overflowing emotions. To my great surprise and admitted relief, the young woman next to me suddenly started sobbing loudly. I hadn't seen her before and didn't know her name. She had long brown hair and wore the short white coat that marked her as a student or first-year resident.

"I'm just the psych intern," she choked out. "I haven't been here very long. My father is sick and I have a test in the fall that I need to study for. He's in California. We don't get along very well." She was crying so hard it wasn't easy to understand her. I looked across the table and noticed the eyebrows of my colleagues all high up on their faces. They looked at this woman with concern, surprise, and some puzzlement. Her comments seemed unexpected, under the circumstances. Janice shifted in her seat and inclined her head. She looked ready to hear more, not entirely certain if she should speak.

From across the table Dr. Berry asked, "Are you . . . ? Have you . . . ? Is your mother . . . ? Is there anyone taking care of your father?" As one of the full-time psychiatrists hired by CSS for our patients, Dr. Berry was responsible for supervising the psych interns who spent time on our service. It amazed me that she could come up with a sensible, focused question when my own mind felt like a jumble of patients' faces and tears.

"No, they're divorced. My sister lives near him and she is seeing him in the hospital. I don't know, I just, I can't, it's so hard . . ." And then she continued sobbing.

Someone reached across the table to her with some tissues which she took and wiped her nose and her eyes. "I haven't seen any patients yet," she said, twisting the tissue in her hands. "I am afraid to see patients who are really sick right now." Some heads nodded around the room.

Gerald, who didn't seem to be able to speak without running his hands through his hair, spoke up. "Gee, uh, well, that is, um, well," and then he turned to Dr. Berry with a look that said "Help!" Gerald recently stepped into the job of office administrator, a large step, as he freely admitted to everyone. He'd previously worked at the clinic as a social worker, but his new role entailed much more responsibility and he wanted to be supportive as well as provide guidance for the staff.

Dr. Berry asked the intern, "Do you think that you need to take a break, perhaps, and maybe not have the pressure of seeing patients for a while?" Gerald nodded along with this question.

The intern said, "Oh, I don't know, I don't know what to do, I am not sleeping and my test is in September."

At this point Janice said, "Do you, I'm sorry, what is your name?"

"Wendy."

"Wendy. Wendy, do you think that the work here might be too difficult for you right now? You have a lot going on in your life. It may be too much to ask."

Wendy wiped her eyes some more and seemed to get herself under control. "I feel guilty about studying when I know my father is sick and then I think that we haven't talked very much in the last ten years but we used to fight all the time and now I know he wishes I were a dermatologist." The laughter at this could have been heard down the hall. Comic relief never seemed so apt a phrase.

Even Wendy managed a smile. "I'm just, I think I need some more sleep and I need to study more even though it is sometimes hard to concentrate." Janice nodded her head as did Dr. Berry.

"Wendy," said Dr. Berry, "why don't we talk after support group and we'll figure out how to make this work for you."

Stan said, "Derm's for wimps," to more laughter around the room.

Wendy blew her nose and the silence returned. This time I didn't feel quite as uncomfortable as everyone sat quietly with their thoughts. And the silence did not last as long.

Briana, a social worker, spoke up and told how she had been on the subway and a panhandler had come through the car announcing that he was hungry. He had AIDS and would someone please give him a dime, nickel, or penny. As he approached she realized it was one of her patients. Most of the people in the room smiled at this. Stan asked if she gave him any money.

"I gave him two dimes and told him to call us for an appointment."

To a chorus of chiding Briana added, "I know. I'm a cheapskate."

"Well, you probably don't get paid that much," added Gerald, looking pointedly at Dr. Jacobs.

Dr. Jacobs had been staring at the floor through much of this, though with a hint of a smile on his face. He now looked up at Gerald and said, "What are you looking at me for? You're the administrator, you give her a raise." We all laughed again, especially Gerald.

# Chapter Two

# 1992  So Much to Learn

The first time I heard about HIV it was called by another name. None of us appreciated then that we were hearing about an illness whose initial impact would be like the earliest shivers and creaks of an earthquake that would shake the entire world.

In the summer of 1982, after my first year of medical school, I met some friends for lunch at my roommate's house in Philadelphia. One of the people there was a fourth-year medical student at a big hospital in New York City. He told us of an illness occurring in gay men that made them very sick and sometimes killed them. No one knew what it was or what caused it. He mentioned that people used the term GRID, which stood for gay-related immune deficiency. The student said that more and more cases of this strange but terrible illness were showing up in other hospitals in New York, and that cases were now being reported in other cities around the country. We talked, that day, of how or why gay men would be victims of a disease like this. From the student's description it sounded scary and ominous.

Within the next two years I'd seen several cases of this illness on my ward rotations. The patients were all young people in their twenties and thirties and they were desperately sick. Some had terrible pneumonia caused by *Pneumocystis*, an organism that had only rarely been seen before. Some patients were covered with purple spots and carried the diagnosis of a sarcoma that was supposed to affect only old men in Greece. Others were just skin and bones, unable to eat, or feverish for reasons that we could not figure out. Gay men made up the majority of our patients, with others being intravenous drug users, both male and female, and the sexual partners of those drug users. In recognition of this broader patient population, the name for the illness became acquired immunodeficiency syndrome (AIDS).

At about this time, in 1984, I heard a lecture by an infectious diseases specialist at the University of Vermont. He spoke of an illness affecting large portions of communities in Central Africa, in Uganda and the Democratic Republic of the Congo, known then as Zaire. It was recognized in Africa as "slim disease" because patients had severe, unremitting diarrhea and could not eat. They became profoundly wasted and after months of sickness they died. A high prevalence of tuberculosis in these regions complicated and generally worsened the course of this illness, which predominantly affected young adults and working-age people. Because the ill could not work and required someone to care for them, economic downturns were becoming apparent in these already impoverished regions. The infectious diseases specialist giving the talk noted the link between "slim disease" and the acquired immune deficiency syndrome, formerly GRID, now being seen in the United States. Research indicated that AIDS and "slim disease" were manifestations of the same condition. Increasing numbers of cases were being diagnosed in the United States, such that by the end of 1984, over seven thousand Americans had died of or were suffering from AIDS.

Before 1981, while I was in college, this illness didn't even exist. Yet by the time I finished medical school and began my training in internal medicine, AIDS patients made up the bulk of cases in many inpatient medical hospital units. The stigma around the disease spread even faster than the disease itself, especially in those early years when the cause was unknown and the effect always devastating. The unknown frightened people. In hospitals, housekeeping services didn't want to clean the rooms of those patients. Wary food service employees left meal trays outside the hospital room doors of patients who were too ill to sit up, much less get out of their beds and walk across the room to the door. Once, during residency, I mentioned AIDS to a colleague as we took the elevator upstairs. The man standing next to me jumped away from me. He looked aghast, as if just hearing the word AIDS might be contagious.

The huge stigma surrounding patients with HIV came from fear of the illness and judgment of the lifestyles of the patients. AIDS was associated with homosexuals and drug addicts. In 1985, when the human immunodeficiency virus was identified, it became clear that virus replicated in white blood cells and therefore could be found in blood and body fluids. AIDS could be transmitted only through blood or through sex. Sharing needles for injection drug use could transmit infection as could exposure through vaginal or anal intercourse. Prostitution became a risk factor for AIDS. Babies were born with the virus from their infected mothers, and hundreds of recipients of blood or blood product transfusions also became sick. Many hemophiliacs became infected before measures were taken to protect the blood supply. Transmission did not occur from hugging or handshakes or toilet seats or breathing the same air. Nonetheless, the stigma of an AIDS diagnosis brought out the worst in people. Doctors and nurses refused to care for HIV-infected patients, employers fired them, families rejected them, and schools expelled them.

And yet many people responded to those in need. The mystery and severity of the illness fascinated some just as it repelled others. Where did it come from? Why now? Why did it progress this way? How could it be stopped? The glaring need for help brought many to the field. Caring for AIDS patients began without guidelines or algorithms, no textbooks or handbooks or cheat sheets. Trying to treat an illness that we didn't understand put us on the very forward edge of medicine. A clear sense of a new frontier existed for those providers drawn to devote themselves to the care and treatment of patients with AIDS.

I grew up in a small college town three hundred miles from New York City. I went to college in New England. A year abroad after high school and several foreign study programs had nurtured in me a love of travel and an interest in other cultures and people. I graduated from medical school in Philadelphia and went back to upstate New York for my residency. My medical education and training corresponded almost exactly with the development of the AIDS epidemic in the 1980s. I remember seeing those first cases as a wide-eyed student, and as a resident I cared for terribly sick AIDS patients in the emergency room, in the intensive care unit, and on the medical wards. It seemed that the patients were all my age. Some were drug addicts, some were hemophiliacs. Many of the male patients were gay.

At first we wore masks, gloves, gowns, hats, and booties, covering ourselves from the unknown threat that lurked somewhere within these horribly sick patients. As we tried to protect ourselves, our costumes dramatically reinforced the patients' sense of fear and isolation. Even after identification of the virus, and knowing the virus couldn't be transmitted casually, admitting offices usually placed hospitalized AIDS patients in rooms by themselves.

The implications of this forced separation always weighed on me. Many of the gay men already struggled with their families over issues of homosexuality. Having a hateful, frightening disease made their situation all the more tragic.

After residency, now thirty years old, I moved to New York City to be with my girlfriend as she completed her own residency program. I worked in a general medical clinic and took care of a lot of middle-aged and elderly men and women who didn't want to take their blood pressure medicine. I eventually wanted to work with underserved populations in Africa or India, and I studied for a master's in public health at Columbia University on what I thought was my way to spending the first part of my career working abroad. AIDS patients came to the ER in the hospital where I worked; they had pneumonia and tuberculosis, brain abscesses and rapidly progressing blindness. A few came to the general medicine clinic, but this occurred less frequently. More often they presented to the emergency room and waited to be admitted, or they stayed sick at home, away from the doctors. No AIDS clinic existed at the time.

A diagnosis of AIDS was considered a death sentence. As a result, many of the people who knew they were at risk did not want to be tested for the virus. They did not want to know, and definitely did not want anyone else to know, that they had HIV. Sometimes people without any risk save their own vulnerability to popular paranoia came to the emergency room thinking they had the virus. They asked for the test, wondering if, on some doorknob or toilet seat, they might have become infected with this strange and deadly disease. Occasionally one of my clinic patients asked to be tested. I had a charming, nearly deaf elderly man from Ukraine who wanted an AIDS test. This took me by surprise, but finding out what led him to ask for the test proved difficult. "Why do you want this test?" I asked him.

He leaned in and cupped one hand behind his ear. "Eh?" He winced as he spoke.

"WHY DO YOU WANT THIS TEST?" I asked again, quite a lot louder.

"AIDS test. Yes." His left hand stayed cupped behind his ear.

"WHY?"

He just nodded at me.

"DO YOU HAVE ANY RISK FACTORS?"

"Eh?"

"RISK FACTORS? FOR AIDS?"

"Eh?"

"DO YOU EVER SLEEP WITH PROSTITUTES?" By this time I was shouting. I almost started laughing, imagining what the secretaries outside my door were thinking. I did send the test. It came back negative.

One of the nurse practitioners I worked with wanted to build up her own panel of patients, but she refused to take on a patient with HIV. Her aversion to "that kind of patient" surprised me a lot. I realized I didn't need to go anywhere far away to take care of an underserved population. Clearly, caring for AIDS patients would expose me to new cultures and people. I felt an urge to reach beyond the clutter of masks and gloves to ease the loneliness of my patients. Besides, I wanted to stay with Shari and we talked of starting a family. I sent my résumé to Dr. Jacobs when I heard about the program at Cornell. In 1992 he called me and offered me a job at CSS. I said yes.

I got to Stewart's room shortly after nine in my second week at CSS.

"Hello, Stewart, how are you this morning?"

"Oh, Dr. Ball, I'm, well, I, what do you think? How am I doing?"

"You are definitely better, but here, put your oxygen back on, here you go. You need to wear this."

"Yes, I know, yes. I am, but I'm, you know, it's just that my breathing, I, it's just that, how am I?"

"You look a little short of breath. Certainly better than before."

"I am. I'm short of breath. But I'm better, right? I still am short of breath. Can you tell me anything? Did you see my chest X-ray?"

"You haven't had an X-ray since yesterday morning. Remember we talked about the results?"

"Yes, no, I mean, yes. You said it was OK. It's just that, it's just that, it's not PCP right? I don't have that. I just have pneumonia, right?"

"I think it is PCP. I can't tell for sure without the bronchoscopy," a procedure he'd so far refused. "But we are treating you as if you have PCP. And you're getting antibiotics for bacterial, regular pneumonia as well."

"So it might not be PCP?"

"Without the bronchoscopy I can't say for sure. We're treating you for both just to be on the safe side."

"It's not something else? I don't have anything else?"

"Do you want something else?"

"No, I mean, you really think it's PCP. You do?"

"Yes, I do."

"But I'm getting better, right? So it might not be PCP. It could be some-thing else. It could just be pneumonia. I could be getting better from some-thing else."

"We really think this is PCP. All your symptoms make us think that's what you have. Your T cells are very low. You haven't been on anything to protect you against PCP. It is possible that you have a different kind of pneumonia, but PCP is at the top of our list. You are getting better; that's good. But you must wear your oxygen."

"But, Dr. Ball, I'm getting better, right? My X-ray is OK? You said my X-ray is OK?"

"Your X-ray is OK. It's not great, it's not worse than before. The X-ray may not improve as quickly as your symptoms do. But yes, I think you are getting better."

"I'm better, right?"

"Yes, Stewart, yes, you're better. Your breathing is better and your fevers have gone. You need to still wear your oxygen, OK? Let me take a listen to you."

Stewart's skin was clammy and his thinning hair stood straight up on his head. A short man with dark brown eyes and an expression of worry that never left his face, Stewart personified anxiety. He relentlessly asked the same questions, interrupted the answers to ask the questions again. He repeated the answers but didn't seem to digest the information; or else, more likely, he wanted a different answer and so asked the question again. I listened and repeated myself and listened and repeated myself. I tried not to get annoyed with him. Sometimes I succeeded. He made me think of Valium, but whether the Valium was for him or for me was not clear.

He leaned forward in his bed as I lifted his damp gown from his back. With my stethoscope I listened to the little crackles his lungs made when he took a deep breath, like the sound in your head when you eat toast. His rate of breathing was slower than the other day when he could barely talk, but still faster than it should be for someone just resting in bed.

PCP. *Pneumocystis* pneumonia, the best known of all the dread diseases associated with AIDS. An opportunistic infection, it was the most frequent index illness in those with HIV who were untreated or unaware of their infec-tion. In the 1980s, before it was recognized that there were treatments to pre-vent the onset of PCP, this pneumonia developed in nearly three quarters of those infected with HIV, and many of those patients died. People still die from PCP, unfortunately. Even today, the occasional patient comes to our emergency department with fever, shortness of breath, and a dry cough. These patients may be unaware of their HIV infection or may not be getting care despite knowing they have the virus. Some patients see the doctor but don't take the medications to suppress HIV and eventually their immune systems falter.

PCP used to stand for *Pneumocystis carinii* pneumonia. It now just stands for *Pneumocystis* pneumonia. Antonio Carinii and Carlos Chagas identified pneumocysts in rats and guinea pigs in the early twentieth century; hence the name. In the 1950s, several cases of PCP among malnourished children in orphanages in Iran marked one of the first documented outbreaks of this illness. In the early 1990s genetic typing recognized that Dr. Carinii's *Pneumocystis carinii* infected only rats and did not infect people. Since 1999 the pneumocyst that infects humans has been recognized as *Pneumocystis jiroveci* (pronounced yee-roh-veet'-zee, after Otto Jiroveci, a Czech parasitologist), but we continue to refer to it as PCP.

Details of nomenclature aside, in 1992 we diagnosed PCP more than any other opportunistic infection associated with HIV and Stewart almost certainly had it. He'd used heroin to soothe his nerves until 1986, when his blood tested positive for HIV and he finally quit drugs. He'd been a patient at our clinic for four years and his T cell count was a very low 25 per cubic milliliter. Prior to his coming to CSS, Stewart had developed a severe allergic reaction to a common antibiotic routinely used to prevent the development of PCP in patients with low T cell counts. He'd been hospitalized for weeks with a life-threatening rash that caused much of his skin to peel off. Stewart had never been a very calm person, and this awful experience popped his anxiety level off the meter. He became caught between his understandable distrust of medications and his terror of dying. This resulted in a hyperattentiveness to any kind of symptom. I knew his phone number by heart from all the times I called him back to hear about his congestion, his cough, the prickly feeling on his right arm, the dry throat, runny nose, loose stool, hard stool, watery eyes, white tongue, feeling of breathlessness, wax in his ears. If ever I offered a treatment or medication for one of his ailments, he asked me dozens of questions about it, asking the same questions over and over. What was the medication? What did it do? It's for my cough. Will it work? What are the side effects? Does it cause a rash? What did it do to other people who took it? It's for a cough. What kind of medication was it? Would the medication help him? And then, since I was suggesting a treatment, he'd ask what the implications were. Would his symptoms get better? Did they mean he was getting worse? I'm not getting worse. Do you think I have AIDS? I do have AIDS. But I'm not worse. I'm not worse? Do I need a test? Do I need another test? Do I need a CT scan? When he ran out of questions he would start the list over and ask the same questions again. I wondered if Valium came in six-packs.

He could become fixated on what I considered a minor symptom and I couldn't always convince him that he didn't need a certain test or intervention, often one a friend or family member recommended. Sometimes the relentless questions wore me down and I ordered tests that might not really be indicated or treatments that could have been avoided. At the same time his anxiety led him to refuse medications or tests that he really needed. The current hospital admission and his refusal to undergo the bronchoscopy exemplified this behavior. Bronchoscopy involves looking at the lungs from the inside with a tiny light at the end of a very tiny flexible tube. Lung fluid can be withdrawn and lung tissue biopsied using the fiber-optic tube. The fluid or the biopsy allows us to make a definitive diagnosis of PCP. Without the bronchoscopy we can only treat PCP presumptively, that is, without certainty. The resident on the pulmonary service who attempted to get Stewart's permission for the procedure gave him an exhaustive explanation of what a bronchoscopy involved. He answered Stewart's questions for twenty minutes, and then Stewart said no. The resident looked as if he needed a stiff drink after that episode. But ultimately, without the information that the procedure could provide, we didn't know if Stewart had PCP. We treated him as if he did, and fortunately he improved.

"What do you hear, Dr. Ball, I'm better, don't you think? Do you think I'm better?"

"I think your lungs sound better. Your fever is down, your oxygenation has improved. This is good."

"So I can go to the bar mitzvah?"

"The what?"

"My nephew, the bar mitzvah in Florida."

"When is the bar mitzvah?"

"Saturday."

"This Saturday?"

"Yeah."

"Is Karen going?"

"My wife?"

"Your wife."

"No, she hates my sister. Just me going."

"You know, this is the first I've heard about a bar mitzvah, but Stewart, today's Thursday. I really don't think it's a good idea to go to Florida on Saturday."

"But I'm better, you said I'm better. I can tell that my fever is down. I think I should be able to, you know, I think I'll be fine."

"The treatment for PCP that you're getting takes twenty-one days. We don't have a definitive diagnosis, but staying here would really be the best thing for you."

"But, Dr. Ball, can't you give me some other medications? Can't I take some pills for this? I'm better. I could take some pills."

"You are somewhat better, yes. But you need a full course of treatment. I can't just let you go to Florida. You're still short of breath, and you're not finished with the treatment."

"But there are pills I can take. I am better, my X-ray is better."

"Stewart, listen. You need to be here. But I can't force you to stay. I really think that you should be in the hospital for the whole medical treatment. I think it's best for you to stay here. If you do go, though, you'll need to sign an AMA form. AMA means 'against medical advice.'"

"My plane is tomorrow afternoon. I'll stay tonight, OK? I can still get IV medication tonight and then go in the morning. That's OK, right?"

"Let's see how you are overnight. Hopefully tomorrow you'll feel even better. But you'll need to sign that AMA paper if you leave tomorrow."

"But you'll give me pills to take? What pills will you give me? Do you think they'll be strong enough? Will they treat PCP if I have it? And I'll take them in Florida. It's my nephew. Karen isn't going, she doesn't like my sister. I said I'd go so it'll be OK. I'm sure I'll be fine there. I'll take the pills."

"Let's see how you are in the morning. We'll talk more then. I'll see you later. Please put your oxygen back on."

I left his room and wondered if I should laugh or cry.

Out in the hall I saw Felicity, the social worker for both Dennis and Stewart, just emerging from another patient's room. A security guard sat in a plastic chair by the door, reading a magazine. I heard Felicity say good-bye and tell the person inside the room that he'd get his old room back as soon as the door was fixed. I concluded that she was visiting Dennis.

"How is he?" I asked.

"Oh, you know, he gets so upset. Now he wants his old room back."

"Is he scary?"

"Well, no, he's much better. I mean he's still a little wild-looking. I think he just gets upset."

"Can I ask you about Stewart?"

"Of course, my dear. How are you, by the way?" Felicity looked at me seriously and nodded her head up and down very firmly a couple of times.

"Thank you, things are OK." I didn't want to think too hard about how to answer that question right then. I was in the middle of rounds; I needed to finish and get back up to my office. I appreciated her asking but held back from offering the jumbled tangle of impressions and feelings that these first weeks had created. "I'm getting into the swing of things," I said.

"Good, that's good, I hope it's not too hard."

We often said that Felicity seemed to have walked out of a previous century. She pinned up her hair in a loose bun with brown wisps falling around her face. She spoke in a soft, whispery voice that never ever reflected anger or even annoyance. She could find something positive or sympathetic to say about the rudest, nastiest, most difficult person, and she often made us laugh at her incredible generosity of spirit to even the most egregious offender. When I first met her I thought she couldn't be real.

"Is Stewart better?" she asked. "I'm going to see him later this afternoon."

"Yes, he's better. Fortunately. But now he's talking about going to the—"

"Bar mitzvah"—we both said it at once.

"Oh, I know. He is so fond of this nephew of his." Felicity brushed back one of her tendrils of hair and with one hand tucked it up into her bun. "He was telling me all about it a few weeks ago."

"Well, I just feel that I can't really let him go. He still needs oxygen. He wants so much to be better and, yes, he's a little better, but, you know, an airplane . . ."

"It's not a good idea."

"No, I really don't think so."

"OK, well, I'll see what he says when I stop by later. I'll reinforce that he should stay." She gave me another one of her firm nods and turned to walk toward the nurses' station in her dark skirt and blue tights and pumps, unsuccessfully trying again to get that stray bit of hair back into her bun. I moved on to the next patient on my rounds.

In the room next to Stewart lay Mr. Torres. Like Stan's patient Edward, Mr. Torres was dying of his illness, and a morphine drip hung from the IV pole next to his bed. I hadn't been on the service long enough to have known him before he went into a coma. Unlike Edward, Mr. Torres had no family who came to visit. A neighborhood priest had come by one day and a sister who lived in Texas had been contacted. She wasn't coming to see him. He had a single room, the bedclothes folded neatly, no cards or flowers, and the shade pulled down. Mr. Torres did not talk or open his eyes. He would wince if you pinched him but otherwise he didn't move spontaneously. He had high fevers and had been receiving a whole slew of antibiotics at one point. Despite our efforts, he was dying. Recently, with the permission of his sister, we had cut back on all the interventions. Some days I spent very little time in his room. I listened to his chest, called his name, squeezed his hand, and left. Some days I sat next to his bed. I felt guilty somehow, either way. If I left quickly, I would tell myself that he wasn't aware of it and it didn't matter. If I sat with him for a little while, I felt guilty that I didn't spend more time or that I couldn't do more for him.

Occasionally, not often enough I'm afraid, I would sit next to him and hold his hand and look at his face. As I write this, I realize that I confuse his face with many other faces over the years. Male, female, old, young, wrinkled, smooth, pale, dark, quiet faces lying there. Sometimes I would sit and hold a hand and look at a face. So many questions run through my mind. What life was there behind those eyes? Was there sadness? Was there love? What was this person like as a small child? Did he or she run and jump into a mother's arms? Did he love to drive fast in a car? Was there violence? Was there jubilation? Sometimes there was part of a history I could guess at. I knew she'd used heroin or that he'd loved the bathhouses. Or I knew that a son came to visit after his shift and would sit where I sat and hold the hand of his mother or his dad.

No one held Mr. Torres's hand. Maybe the nurse did, I don't know. Sometimes when I sat there I tried not to ask questions in my mind, tried not to think about my day or my next patient. I just sat quietly. I tried to convey to Mr. Torres that he was not alone. I didn't know him, I hadn't known him prior to his being in a coma; I didn't know his life. It didn't feel right calling him by his first name, Emiliano. I didn't even know the sound of his voice. We might not get along if we knew each other. He might be a lout or a creep. Sometimes I wondered if I was intruding, if I had a right to be there. I was trying to give him something; I was thinking about him, caring about him in the extremely limited way that I could care for this man whom I didn't know. I was recognizing him, his life, and his passage out of life, so I felt that it was OK to be there. As a doctor I offered no cure, no turnaround of the deadly infection that he carried. As a person, as a fellow traveler in this crazy world, I offered a few moments of companionship on the last part of his life journey.

Maybe no one had ever sat quietly with him. And maybe he never would have wanted anyone to. But I felt it was important to acknowledge him. No matter who he was or had been, I was there as a witness to this moment in his life. I know that I got more than I gave in those moments. It seemed that his life would end and no one would know, no one would cry. It felt lonely in his room. Eventually I got up and went out into the bright hall, leaving him alone again, lying on the bed in the low-lit room behind me.

Back up on the twenty-fourth floor at CSS, the day's clinic ended at four and we gathered in the conference room for team rounds. We had these rounds every day after clinic as part of our multidisciplinary approach to patient care. All the patients, outpatients seen that day, were discussed and all the providers, including the nurses and social workers, attended. Dr. Jacobs came to team rounds upstairs once a week because he saw patients at CSS on Wednesdays. Once a week, on Fridays, we had rounds for the inpatients downstairs in the hospital with the floor nurses.

I sat down at the big conference table as Gerald called the first patient.

"Kevin was here today," Stan said, sighing. "Kevin was not in a very good mood, something that's not very surprising, although I confess I continue to hope for miracles, atheist that I am. He continues to be angry about me not giving him DDI after he developed pancreatitis from it last year. He blames me for his getting pancreatitis, but he wants me to prescribe DDI for him again despite my many efforts to explain that I don't want him to have pancreatitis." Stan sighed again. "He gets right up in my face and says, 'So I'm just supposed to *DIE*?' And then I try to calm him down and assure him that he is not going to die. He's on Zidovudine and his T cells have gone up a little. He's had some thrush recently and I gave him some more Diflucan and ordered labs for him."

"I saw Kevin too. He's still mad at you," said Briana, looking at Stan. "His roommate was in a car accident with Kevin's car so he wanted to know if I would call his car insurance company. He wasn't happy when I said no."

"He yelled at the front desk again," added Mary Rose, one of our nurses. "He was really nasty. Should he see psych?"

Stan laughed and looked at Dr. Berry. "Think you can fix him?"

"Oh sure," she said. "Send him to me."

"He won't go," said Stan, shaking his head. "I've suggested it in the past but that didn't go over very well."

"You mean you brought up a psych referral for his anger management?"

"No, I brought it up to suggest that he needed help adjusting to his HIV diagnosis."

"That's a good idea. What did he say?"

"Fuck you."

Everyone laughed, including Stan. "No, I'm kidding, he didn't really say that. He just blew it off, but maybe I'll try to bring it up again with him."

"Anyway," said Briana, "he has active Medicaid and he gets food stamps and spends a lot of time with his sister and her family in Brooklyn."

In these team rounds we reported on our own patients and we heard about everyone else's. Rounds allowed us each to learn who was sick, whose phone had been cut off, who swore at the nurses in the lab, who needed to see the nutritionist. Some patients were known because of how ill they were and how frequently they came to the clinic. Some were known because of their unique personalities, their propensity for causing trouble, or their charming or crazy adventures. In rounds I could express my pleasure at a patient's improvement, my frustration at an ambulette service arriving two hours late, my worry about the abusive husband, or concern over the persistent weight loss. I heard about Maggie's hour-long appointment with her patient as he dealt with putting his dog to sleep, Briana getting her patient to bring in his phone bills, Zoe Prin's tense episode with the patient for whom she refused to renew the Valium. My own visit with a patient might have been routine and straightforward, but the social worker could reveal that the patient's husband went back to jail and they were now threatened with eviction. The patient might tell me that she had been clean for three weeks but tell Dr. Berry that she was on a crack binge this past weekend. A day never passed when I didn't hear something unexpected, outrageous, unbelievable, or simply funny about one or more of the patients or their providers. Over time we got to know all the people who came to CSS.

Of course we didn't get to know only the patients. Inevitably we learned about one another. Who was shy, who was funny, who was uncomfortable, and who was overwhelmed. I knew which social worker got right to the point and which one dragged out each sentence without saying much at all. I learned that Mary Rose fell asleep nearly every day in rounds and Randall, another social worker, let slip that he had fantasies about one of the handsome residents. I remember well sitting at that table in one of my first team rounds when I heard Stan swear. He was leaning way back in his padded leather chair, and when the patient's name was called he looked at the ceiling and said,

"He's driving me out of my fucking mind!" I didn't know the patient at the time but clearly everyone else in the room did. They were howling, I mean *howling* with laughter. I knew Stan to be warm, caring, compassionate, and completely professional. His comment surprised me, but it pleased me as well for it revealed a refreshing honesty. I remember at the time thinking, this job is going to be different.

Our clinic prided itself on its multidisciplinary approach to patient care, and the patients clearly benefited from the communication among providers. For a disease that was so hard to treat, this combined approach improved patient care and served as one of the few bright stars in the dark sky of AIDS. Though sometimes rounds seemed overly long or tedious, we all realized how much everyone, ourselves included, benefited from this hour spent together every day.

Next on the list was Lenny, a patient of Maggie's who lived in a men's shelter not far from the hospital. A very likeable fellow, Lenny got along with most of the CSS staff. He had a history of substance use and now struggled, sometimes unsuccessfully, to stay away from cocaine. Maggie had seen him in her office and reported that he was stable with a T cell count in the three hundreds. She'd counseled him about his ongoing intermittent drug use.

Mary Rose reported that Lenny had been very animated in the lab when he went to get his blood drawn. Showing off a new pair of pants, he said he'd found them in the Dumpster on First Avenue, a few blocks from the hospital. White pants, practically new. Mary Rose kept a straight face up until that point but now she started laughing. " 'Check it out!' he said to me, and he was so proud of his new pants. They were nice-looking pants, white with pockets. They looked like house officer pants, you know, the pants that the interns wear sometimes."

Someone said, "Uh-oh."

Mary Rose laughed again. " 'And look, there's even a doctor's name in the waistband,' so he shows me and the name in his pants is Zoe Prin, MD."

Everyone burst out laughing. Zoe, clearly mortified, couldn't help but smile at the idea that Lenny had pulled her pants out of the Dumpster and worn them to clinic. "I was cleaning out my closet!" she said defensively. "I didn't want to give them to the Salvation with my name in them."

"So you threw them away?"

"They are perfectly good. Lenny loves them!" Mary Rose added.

"He should; they were practically new."

"You never wore them?"

"Well, maybe once or twice."

Stan asked Zoe what else she'd cleaned out of her closet. "Maybe I should go out and check that Dumpster."

Gerald looked at Stan skeptically. "I think Zoe's pants would be a bit small for you."

# Chapter Three

# 1992 No Easy Answers and Little to Offer

"I ain't takin' that shit. No way. No way."

Peaches sat across the desk from me slouched in her chair with her thick dark hair standing up in various directions on her head. She had straightened it at some point in the past but it hadn't been brushed recently. She wore a yellow oversized man's shirt, her large abdomen stretching the fabric. She absently scratched at the rash on her belly at the opening where a button was missing. Her face looked lumpy and red with more of the same rash: irritated and itchy, and she had clearly been scratching. She gave one of the raucous laughs that always made me smile. A laugh that made her belly shake. "Dr. Ball, you know that shit kills people."

I resisted the urge to put my head face down on the desk and bang my fist on the table. In 1992 we were still years away from effective treatment for HIV. "That shit" was basically one of only two medicines I had to offer for this disease, and only a few weeks into my job I already knew painfully well how little good they did. Many of my patients knew it, too. In this case, "that shit" was AZT (short for 3′-azido-3′-deoxythymidine, also known as zidovudine). Originally developed in the 1960s as an anti-leukemia agent, AZT was pulled from the shelf and dusted off in the mid-1980s along with many other drugs to assess their efficacy in halting, slowing, or somehow inhibiting HIV.

In 1987 the Food and Drug Administration (FDA) approved the use of AZT in patients with HIV after a study showed that CD4 (T cell) counts improved in significantly more patients who took it than in those who didn't. As the first drug approved for use in the treatment of AIDS, AZT effectively interrupted a certain process in the life cycle of HIV by inhibiting an enzyme known as a reverse transcriptase. At the time, although we understood AZT's mechanism of action, we were unable to directly measure the drug's impact on the amount of virus in the blood. As a surrogate marker, rising T cells meant better immunity, fewer opportunistic infections. AZT didn't necessarily make anyone actually feel better, however.

The approval of AZT met with a divided reception. Some felt that the drug had not been adequately studied or that the purported positive effects were exaggerated and misleading. Others accused the manufacturer of being coldhearted and calculating, interested only in cashing in on others' misfortune by rushing to market an inadequate, indeed a potentially toxic, medication. But patients had been dying of AIDS for six years; for many doctors and patients AZT was a first ray of light in a very dark tunnel. Although it was far from a cure, its release to the public was met with jubilation by many.

When I first started working at CSS, I found that some patients were anxious to take anything I prescribed, anything that stood even a remote chance of slowing down what the AIDS virus was doing to them. But I also had skeptical patients whose hesitation stemmed from a variety of reasons. Some already led lives in chaos from poverty or violence or drugs; their illness presented just another lousy hand from a deck stacked against them. Other patients were fearful, overwhelmed by their diagnosis, and worried that medicine would only make things worse. Finally, there were those who bought into the thinking that AIDS was a conspiracy, a government-manufactured plot to get rid of homosexuals and drug addicts; that or a vaccine study gone hopelessly haywire, with unsuspecting Africans the initial human guinea pigs.

Peaches got her data from the street, and the street did not like AZT. Too many side effects, too many dead friends. It didn't help for me to point out that by the time some patients started taking AZT, their disease had advanced too far to be turned around or stopped; it usually wasn't AZT that killed those friends. For the most part people tolerated the drug, but it could cause low blood counts in some patients and severe muscle aches in others. Most patients got a headache the first few times they took it. In addition, when it first came on the market, AZT had to be taken every four hours around the clock. Patients needed to set their alarms to wake up and take their pills.

Though it was the first and for a while the only medication against the virus, it wasn't enough. It quickly became clear that AZT did not produce any miracles. The next drug, didanosine, didn't help much either. Patients on either one saw their T cells go up for a while, but before long they were on their way back down. It was like using a peashooter with soggy peas against a charging wild boar. Peaches wasn't going to take "that shit." I could write her a prescription, and she might even fill it and bring the pills home. But given her comments in my office, I could bet that she wouldn't take them. We needed more effective treatment.

Once, before I came to CSS, I cared for an elderly Russian lady who had terribly high blood pressure. She would come into my office and wave a much-handled paperback drug compendium at me. "Side effects!" she'd yell. "You give me this drug and it has so much side effects!" She was about four and a half feet tall with enormous glasses and long, wild-looking brown hair. She wore huge gray orthopedic shoes. We would go over the side effects of the diuretic or the beta-blocker and she resisted my every suggestion. I could not make her see that just because a side effect was listed in her book, it didn't mean that it would happen to her. "But you don't know, do you?" she'd ask me, her eyes hugely magnified behind her glasses. I couldn't convince her that the medication would not cause a seizure or hemolytic anemia or a total body rash or muscle aches or any one of the hundreds of possible side effects listed in that compendium of hers. Her resistance to my recommendations exasperated me. She charmed me, however, with her great stories, her thick accent, and the way she inevitably tried to slip me a five-dollar bill at the end of each appointment. I learned from her feistiness and her arguments that just because I wore a white coat, my patients weren't going to do everything I asked. I had to come up with better means of persuasion. It didn't take me long as a doctor to realize that when a patient had misgivings about or fear of a medication, it was highly likely that the patient wouldn't take it consistently. In 1992 I didn't know how much time and energy would one day be spent on getting AIDS patients to take their medications. I just wished we had one that worked.

Peaches missed many of her appointments. She and her four young boys lived in a drug-infested building. The boys had been taken from her when her drug screen tested positive after the birth of her youngest. She went to a rehabilitation facility for several months to get clean and she worked hard to satisfy the officials in order to get her children back. She mostly steered clear of drugs now but admitted with a grin that sometimes the neighbors lured her into smoking crack with them late at night. She'd need to sleep on the couch most of the next day while a home attendant got the boys ready for school.

I asked Peaches if this happened very often.

"Now don't get all funny on me, Dr. Ball. I'm clean. I want to stay clean. But those guys—" and in a sing-song voice she crooned, "Peeeeeeeee-ches," and she started laughing in a way that made me smile. "They tempt me, damn it, and I say no, no, no, but sometimes I'm just out there for five minutes for just one hit." Her belly jiggled with her laughter and she scratched herself again. I liked her straightforward simplicity. She didn't make up stories or tell me only what she thought I wanted to hear. She loved her boys and had her weaknesses. The father of her third son had died of AIDS. Fortunately, none of the boys were infected. I worried about what would happen to those boys if Peaches's HIV continued to go untreated.

Support group met twice a month. It was already quiet when I tiptoed in, a few minutes late after seeing Peaches. Dr. Jacobs sat in his usual chair against the wall and I could feel the quiet like a heavy cloud. Janice smiled a hello from her place at the head of the table. My leather chair made the only noise, creaking as I sat down. I looked around and saw most everyone staring at the table. A few people sat outside the circle of the table and they, like Dr. Jacobs, stared at the floor. The silence went on and on, like the held breath of the crowd before the maestro raises his baton. These silent moments always seemed so full of focus, each person concentrating on his or her own thoughts, own ache. I found myself reviewing the patients I had seen that day in clinic or my list of patients downstairs on the inpatient unit. I allowed myself to think of their families, the people who loved them, their children or their parents, how much pain this disease was causing. I often felt tearful and overwhelmed as I sat there. I knew that the people around the table were all thinking similar thoughts, and although the silence could seem awkward, it felt communal. In that room with my colleagues, even if we didn't speak, the collective sense of being in this together eased the individual heartache that came from our work. The idea of actually talking about any of that to the assembled crowd seemed like jumping on the table naked: so vulnerable, so exposed.

Janice usually allowed the silence to continue until someone spoke. Occasionally she asked what the feeling in the room was that day. Today the silence continued for minutes on end.

Felicity finally said, "I just wanted to say thank you to Anna, who covered me last week when I was out." Felicity nodded her head emphatically up and down, escaping wisps of brown hair waving around. "I know that it wasn't an easy week with Humphrey dying." Anna looked up and acknowledged the thanks as Felicity turned to Maggie. "Maggie, how are you doing? I know that Tom is quite sick."

"Tom-Tom," Maggie said, and her eyes filled with tears. She studied the table for a moment as they trickled down her cheeks. She tried to smile and brushed at them with the back of her hand. "Well, he has been getting worse. Before it was pneumonia and then the diarrhea and then the stroke."

"This is your patient?" asked Janice. "Tom-Tom?"

Maggie smiled. "Yes, that's what I call him. He's such a sweet guy. He's not doing well at all. His lover, Roddo, is my patient, too."

"It sounds like it's pretty painful for you."

Felicity still looked at Maggie, nodding her head up and down with a serious expression.

"I'm very attached to both of them. Maybe too attached, I don't know. I know what's going to happen. I'm spending so much time with them both, but Tom-Tom is still in the hospital."

I knew from Stan that Maggie spent nearly an hour each day at Tom's bedside. The two men had become personal friends of Maggie's; they'd all had dinner together and been to each other's apartments. Maggie had her own nicknames for Rodney and his lover, pet names. At CSS a particularly notorious patient would earn a nickname, such as Mr. Charming for the man who swore at the front desk, or Joe Testosterone for the patient who constantly asked for more testosterone. The pet names Maggie used for her patients rarely became nicknames used by the other CSS staff. Maggie's involvement with her patients at times became too personal. As with Tom and Rodney, she occasionally crossed some invisible border that separated the patients and physicians in our clinic. I could understand how this happened in an environment such as ours. We saw patients in our offices or in their beds in the hospital; often they'd been rejected by their families or their sources of emotional support. Sometimes the entire family was rejected by a community because the son or husband or mother had a diagnosis of AIDS. The patients and their families instead became a part of a community at CSS, taken in by the doctors, nurses, social workers, chaplain, and psychiatrists. This brought an intensity to our work that sustained us. The stigma and sadness and death could burn us out though, in ways we couldn't entirely prepare for or prevent. We had to protect ourselves and remember our roles as providers, because the patients needed us to be there for them as professionals.

Maggie said, "I think Roddo's really going to take it hard if Tom-Tom dies."

I could see that Maggie would take it hard as well.

We spent lots of time with our patients; it was impossible not to become personally involved. Sometimes, especially with this disease, it seemed the only thing we *could* offer was a held hand or a few minutes to sit quietly at the bedside and listen. Naturally we developed attachments. In the support group with Janice, we got to let down our guard a bit and feel the emotion of the moment. Compassion united all of us in that room. As professionals we each worked hard to maintain an appropriate balance in our relationships with our patients, a balance that allowed us to care deeply and still maintain our effectiveness and objectivity.

When I was a little girl, the doctor in our town made house calls. We lived in a village in the farmlands of upstate New York. We really did call it a village. Dr. Benton came to our house in his big green car and had a classic black bag with a lot of clinking bottles and packages in it. When I had strep throat he came and sat on my bed and took my temperature, looked at my throat with his special light, and listened to my chest with his stethoscope. He'd come in the late afternoon or in the evening, after office hours, which took place downstairs in his big house in town. He drove all over that hilly country seeing a sick kid like me and the old farmer's wife with diabetes and the local butcher at home with a broken ankle and anybody else in his practice who couldn't make it in to see him that day. He wasn't the only doctor in town, but I know the two or three others also made their house calls. We took these visits for granted, but by the time I was in college and heading for medical school, the house call had become the exception instead of the rule.

Those doctors making their house calls in small towns knew their patients in ways that most doctors no longer do. The doctor was a part of the community; he knew the family, the smell of the kitchen, the ruts in the driveway, and the number of dogs tied up in the backyard. Severe illness took its toll on everyone, not just the patient. The doctor was a piece of all of this, a part of the fabric of the community. A death might hit everyone hard and be shared, or a death might be a welcome respite for patient and family. At CSS our ability to care for such a desperately sick group of people depended on the sanity and support that we provided for one another. And while we created for the patients a safe place away from the shame and stigma that surrounded AIDS, we understood that the providers and the patients had different roles, needs, and purposes. No one said, "Don't get involved," but we knew that blurring the lines between work and personal involvement could be perilous.

"I don't know," said Mary Rose. "I think we all take it hard when a patient dies. I'm not the doctor, Maggie, and I know you care a lot about all of your patients. But we may only see them in the lab. We talk to them and tell jokes to get them to relax when we draw their blood. We see them a lot. But then suddenly they're gone. It's hard." Her voice drifted off. Heads around the room nodded.

Mary Rose worked three days a week at CSS as one of our part-time nurses. Her husband was a policeman on Long Island where they lived with their three daughters. Mary Rose didn't put up with any bullshit from the patients. She yelled at them when they were late or lost their prescriptions. She harangued people to quit smoking or stop doing crack. She had a huge heart and spent lots of time talking with patients, asking them about their lives, offering support and encouragement. Mary Rose didn't often come to support group because she had Thursdays off. Today when she spoke up, she too had tears in her eyes.

Maggie looked sadly at Mary Rose.

"Mary Rose, are you talking about Tom?" Janice asked.

"No, no. I mean yes, I'm sad to know that Tom's so sick. He and Rodney are so funny together and I'm sad for them both. And for you, Maggie. But so much happens away from this place, in the hospital or wherever, that we don't know about. Suddenly the person isn't there anymore and we don't get a chance to really process it. We don't even *know* about it."

Nods and silence around the table; people were looking at Maggie and Mary Rose.

"It's true. At least you guys know when you're sending a patient to a nursing home." This time Suzette spoke up and she looked at Stan and then at me. "You know pretty well that you're never going to see them again. We're over here with the outpatients and we might not have any idea what's going on over on the floor. It's rare we get a chance to think that this is the last time we'll see someone. Although with the way some people look, we might wonder sometimes." Suzette was our head nurse and although younger than Mary Rose, she'd been with Dr. Jacobs from the time when CSS was a one-room operation in a random hallway in the hospital. She knew every patient, knew their medications and their allergies, their home life, their habits. She practically knew their phone numbers. She could be very tough, but she had tremendous compassion along with an unflinching work ethic. She made sure the place ran smoothly, and Dr. Jacobs confirmed her importance by referring to her as "Boss." Suzette also had a great sense of humor, a mandate at this job, as I had come to realize.

"The other night when I went home I just couldn't get out of my head the picture of Humphrey in his wheelchair. He looked so bad." Mary Rose looked down at the table as she spoke. "I was thinking that I probably wasn't going to see him again. I drove home and I pulled up in my driveway and my neighbor was in her yard watering some flowers or something, I don't even know what. She waved all friendly and came over to say hello. She's a nice lady, we're friendly, our kids are friends and everything. But when she came over to the car she asked me how was work and she was asking like it was funny, like 'How was your day today, dear?'"

A couple of people around the table groaned.

"I just looked at her and I said, well, the day was not good. One of the patients is dying. 'Dying,' said my neighbor. 'Dying, from AIDS?' So I said, yeah, dying from AIDS."

"And my neighbor backed away from the car and got this really weird expression on her face. It wasn't like she was sad or feeling sorry. She looked, she looked, I don't know, disgusted or creeped out. So then I said, he is a really nice man, you would have liked him. And I felt really mad. She said something like, well, that must be hard and have a good night or something and she practically ran back over to her house."

We were all looking at Mary Rose as she told this story. It was easy to picture the neighbor's face.

No one said anything for a moment. "A lot of people don't understand," said Janice.

"Well, where I live people just don't know. I get home sometimes and I think I'm somewhere so far away. People have no idea."

"Oh, they just have no idea," said Anna.

"Humphrey, he was a sweetie."


Hours later I stood smoking a cigar in a very noisy bar. It tasted terrible. Ten of my colleagues sat at a big table drinking beer. Dr. Berry stood next to me drinking her second martini and smoking a cigarette. We all joked about the fact that none of us smoked "in real life" but there we were. Stan and Molly, one of the social workers, puffed on big stogies, across the room, deep in conversation. Stan's wife sat nearby talking with Felicity. Dr. Berry and I were talking together about support group and how unusual it was to have a group for providers across all of the disciplines. Having never participated in such a thing before, I didn't have any notions of protocol for it. Dr. Berry explained that usually there were separate groups for the nurses or the social workers or the doctors but not all mixed together. We both agreed that it seemed logical to support one another as a team since we all worked as a team. Dr. Berry credited Dr. Jacobs for coming up with that idea and seeing it through. Dr. Jacobs, meanwhile, sat at another part of the table talking with Suzette and two of the social workers. He wore a suit and a dark bow tie and held a cigar in one hand and a beer in the other. He smiled and tipped his head back laughing at something Suzette said.

Since it was a karaoke bar an interesting assortment of music played overhead, from show tunes to heavy metal. Molly's brother, who had come to the bar with her, was a member of a rock band of some renown. Together they sang a Dolly Parton song and Stan and a few others sang "Ramblin' Man." Dr. Jacobs didn't sing. One of the other customers gave a truly awful rendition of "My Way" and we winced politely. Toward the end of the evening the CSS group en masse sang "Love Shack." I looked to find something meaningful in this and I suppose it's true that the song described a big wild party taking place down at the end of a long country road away from everything. I'd known my colleagues for only a few months but I sensed a connection that felt true and right. Shared goals, shared commitment, shared understanding. We trusted one another. We were on this journey together, traveling on a long country road. It felt good to go and have a couple of beers in a karaoke bar.

In the morning I went to see John of the immaculate manicure. My morning messages indicated that he'd been admitted the night before. I'd seen his X-rays and knew that he had a collapsed lung and now had a chest tube in place to re-expand the lung. Having seen the films, I felt pretty certain that he'd been admitted with another case of PCP.

I read through the chart and couldn't find any documentation of the chest tube placement procedure. I couldn't tell when the chest tube had gone in or who had done it or what medications John had been given. The nurses' notes said that the surgeons were with the patient putting the tube in but I saw no note from the surgeons themselves. This was a problem. Any procedure done on a patient in the hospital needed to be documented in the progress notes of the hospital chart. Not just for legal purposes, notes constitute an integral part of patient care. We look to the chart to understand what has happened and the plans for the patient's progress and treatment. Lack of documentation meant sloppy medicine. I contacted the cardiothoracic resident on call to see if he or she had any information.

"Oh, the AIDS guy? Yeah, we put in his chest tube in the ER last night."

"There's no note in the chart."

"Oh, well, we were busy."

"But there's no documentation that the patient even has a chest tube."

"Well, he's an AIDS patient. I mean, we were really busy."

"I understand that you guys are very busy."

"Someone'll come by later and write a note."

"Are you going to follow him?"

"What?"

"Is your service going to follow him to take care of the chest tube?"

"Yeah, sure, someone'll be by later."

"That would be great, thank you."

When I went to see him, I found John of the immaculate manicure sitting up in bed with a thin oxygen tube looped over his ears and beneath his nose. He looked tired but comfortable. His full head of gray hair had been elegantly brushed. I asked him how he'd gotten to the emergency room last night.

"I was watching TV, and then I noticed that it was much harder to breathe." He needed to take a breath to complete this sentence.

"Had your breathing been fine?"

"Well, I noticed that it was a little worse this last week." As he said this he adjusted his nasal oxygen tube with one of those marvelously manicured hands.

"How?" I asked. "In what way? Were you getting out of the house and doing your usual routine?"

"Well, no, I guess not. I wasn't really going out much."

"When did you stop going out?"

"Well, when I got home after the last time I was really pretty good and I went to the store and everything, but in the last few weeks I guess I was slowing down a bit more."

"You went home, when, it was in September, right? And then you missed your appointment with me at the end of the month."

"My sister was visiting. I'm sorry about that. I meant to call and reschedule."

"Don't worry. So now it's five weeks or so since your discharge. How long has it been since you were going out at all?"

"Oh, it's been a few weeks." Somehow at the mention of the word "sister" I thought of Stewart and his bar mitzvah. Stewart would call for a runny nose while John couldn't breathe for weeks but didn't call me.

"I didn't go to my friend's birthday dinner." He paused for a moment and I watched his chest rise and fall. "That was a disappointment but they brought me a big food basket afterwards." He described a big basket with his hands.

"Have you been taking the Dapsone?"

"Yes."

"Have you been short of breath or coughing? Is that what was keeping you from going out?"

"Yes," he said, taking a breath. "It wasn't that obvious I guess, but it was becoming a chore to do anything. I just got my friends to do the shopping and I didn't think about it that much. I wasn't coughing, though, no. Not until a few days ago."

"Fevers?"

"Sometimes fevers, I think. I don't take my temperature usually." A little wave of his hand, a negating gesture.

"And so, what happened last night?"

"Well, I was sitting and watching TV with my friend Roger, and my breathing seemed just worse." John paused and took a few shallow breaths, put his hand on his chest. "I was feeling like I couldn't really breathe right and I began to feel frightened so I had Roger bring me here in a taxi."

I looked at John and watched as he breathed in and out, trying to keep his mouth closed to make the most of the nasal oxygen tube. Had John thought the breathing would just somehow, *poof*, get better? Why hadn't he come in sooner? "Did you have any pain?"

"No, no pain. Well, not until they put the tube in. Wow, that was terrible."

"You mean in the emergency room?"

"Yeah, the surgeons came and they had this tube to put in because they told me that my lung had collapsed," he paused for air, "and they had the nurse give me a shot, but they didn't even wait one minute before they went ahead with that tube. It was really painful."

"Oh, John, I'm so sorry that happened to you."

"That was awful." John shook his head and breathed several breaths in through his nose, as if to suck more oxygen out of the little clear tube. He gracefully adjusted his oxygen again. "They seemed so, so, like I was bothering them. And they were kind of rough and not at all friendly and of course I was thinking, oh, it's because I have AIDS."

"Listen, that is terrible. No one should have that procedure without waiting for the pain medication to take hold. Their service is very busy, it's true, and they are running all over the hospital with all kinds of stuff. I doubt they even had a clue about the HIV and that shouldn't matter anyway. There's no excuse for being rude to you. I'm really sorry that you had that experience." I thought John might be correct in thinking the rudeness and the AIDS were connected, especially after my conversation with the resident. I felt ashamed that someone would treat my patient that way.

"Well, I'm much better now and it doesn't hurt very much. I know they are very busy and at least it was quick. The nurses here are friendly with me."

"Well that's good. I'm glad of that, at least."

I could feel my hands trembling in anger as I left John's room. Later that afternoon I wrote a letter to the head of the hospital and to the head of the cardiothoracic surgery department. I complained about the rude and unprofessional manner in which my patient had been treated, and I complained about the lack of any documentation in the chart.

Some weeks later I got a call from the secretary of the relatively new chairman of the department of cardiothoracic surgery. She said that Dr. Isher would like to meet with me to discuss my letter. I went to the appointment with some apprehension. I felt justified in what I had said in the letter but here I was in a chairman's office. I was an assistant professor, a young attending physician at our big, prestigious hospital. Aware of my lowly status, I wondered if I'd overstepped some line.

Dr. Isher greeted me with a firm handshake. My father always taught me to shake people's hands firmly and to look them in the eye. Dr. Isher's strong grip and warm gray eyes looking into mine put me immediately at ease. He told me that he had read my letter and reviewed John's case with the residents and the fellow involved at the time. Dr. Isher apologized to me and said that even though not everyone felt comfortable taking care of patients with AIDS, it was the responsibility of all of us as physicians to give every patient good care. He also noted the importance of documenting every procedure. While he acknowledged that the cardiothoracic residents could have an overwhelming workload at times, he said that if I ever found a procedure not documented again I should call him immediately.

I left Dr. Isher's office feeling that I had done the right thing to write to him. It didn't change the shoddy care that his residents had given my patient, but it gave me some hope that with Dr. Isher as their model, those residents might offer better care to the next AIDS patient who came their way.

What a time it was in the late 1980s and early 1990s. Stigma, fear, and prejudice surrounded AIDS patients in the non-medical community and the same feelings lurked under the surface in many aspects of their medical care as well. We had been dealing with this disease for more than ten years. Nonetheless, there persisted some very deeply entrenched biases against the disease and those who carried it. City and public hospitals had long been dealing with large numbers of AIDS patients, but private hospitals, even big teaching hospitals, had been almost aggressive in their reluctance to admit these patients. It wasn't until Congress passed the Ryan White Act in 1990 that money became available to hospitals and clinics to provide care for patients with AIDS. Soon we were seeing all kinds of facilities for AIDS patients. It's cynical but true to say that money can definitely improve an institution's sense of altruism. The benefit of meeting and addressing the needs of people with HIV and AIDS far outweighed the hypocrisy of welcoming patients who had previously been shunned. My hospital was no different and followed along with everyone else in supporting the creation of an HIV clinic. We were lucky to have Dr. Jacobs be the one to start the Center for Special Studies. Under his leadership we provided the best care possible, regardless of a patient's illness, background, or ability to pay.

In a teaching hospital the behavior and approach of the residents reflected the attitudes of the senior staff. Some services notoriously lacked support for our patients. The surgical services could be particularly problematic, especially ear, nose, and throat and neurosurgery, delaying needed biopsies or surgery because of fear of infection or pure distaste for the clientele. One head of department reportedly stood up in a grand rounds presentation and announced to the audience that "these patients get what they deserve." If the leadership didn't advocate for our patients, those lower down in the hierarchy could be negatively influenced to follow that example.

Fortunately, the majority of doctors focused on giving our patients the care that they required. While some residents blindly assumed the attitudes of those biased senior attendings, most had gone to school during the earliest days of HIV and they knew the risks as well as the importance of treating all patients the same. It was understood that a person could be infected and not know it. It was understood that you had to wear gloves to draw *everyone's* blood, whether or not they might have HIV. I often felt proud of how well our residents cared for our patients. But sometimes negative attitudes prevailed.

Dr. Isher's care for our patients was exemplary to the point of being noble. A couple of years after my meeting with Dr. Isher, Dr. Jacobs had an HIV-positive patient who required a heart valve replacement. The patient's HIV had not made him sick, he'd not had any complications, and other than his heart valve, he was in good shape. The attending surgeon consulted for the surgery refused to take the case. The story went that this surgeon had remarked to his office nurses that because of the HIV the patient was going to die anyway, so what was the point in putting a whole operating room of staff at risk by operating on him? When Dr. Jacobs heard about it he was livid. He was extremely clear on this issue. What was best for the patient was what needed to be done and this patient needed his heart valve replaced. Dr. Jacobs called the head of cardiothoracic surgery, Dr. Isher. The next day Dr. Isher did the case in the operating room and the surgeon who'd refused scrubbed in to assist him. The patient did well and recovered fully from his surgery. No one in the operating room contracted HIV from operating on him. The surgeon who'd refused to operate did not stay on the hospital staff.

John of the immaculate manicure improved steadily, and the cardiothoracic surgeons took out his chest tube a few days after they put it in. They eventually left a note in the chart, but because the handwriting was so terrible no one could read what it said.

# Chapter Four

# 1994 Too Many Drugs, No Medication

"Hank, are you in here?"

"Just a minute," came his voice from the bathroom. I waited, standing near his empty bed. The other patient in the darkened room lay in the next bed facing away from me toward the lowered blinds. I heard the sink running.

"Hank?"

"Just a minute, I'll be right out."

The bathroom door opened, and with the bright light shining behind him he appeared to be walking out of a spaceship, like E.T. But Hank was no short, shuffling alien. Hank reminded me of Ichabod Crane, all elbows and knees and long legs. Today, as my eyes adjusted to the light, I saw that he wore nothing on his tall, lanky frame other than a long stream of toilet paper inexpertly wrapped around his penis and trailing down his legs. He also had wads of toilet tissue stuffed in his ears and in his nostrils. He moved toward me slowly, as if weary, the toilet paper fluttering along behind him. In the dim light I couldn't make out his face as he ambled past me and sat down on his bed.

"Um . . ." I found it hard to think of anything to say. "Um . . . Hank? What are you doing?"

"I was bleeding."

"You were bleeding from all those places?"

"Can I get some pain medication please?"

"Hank, where is your gown? Why are you naked like this?"

I saw his hospital gown lying crumpled on the bed and I went over and picked it up and held it out to him to put on. He held up his arms and put them into the armholes of the gown. I pulled it up around his shoulders and reached behind him to tie the strings behind his neck. I couldn't see blood anywhere on him.

"I really need some more morphine, Dr. Ball."

I stood back to answer him. He looked tired but did not appear to be in pain. He'd walked across the room without limping or wincing. "Where are you having pain?"

"I was having bleeding from my penis."

"When did that happen?"

"They put a catheter in when I was in the emergency room and when they took it out there were drops of blood."

"What about your ears and your nose? Why do you have this tissue paper all over?"

"I need some more morphine."

Hank had sandy straight hair, pale blue eyes, and a long, smooth jaw. He often had the air of a tall, skinny puppy about him. The toilet paper stuffed into his ears and his nostrils made it look as if he might be preparing for some kind of ritualistic cosmetic surgery.

Just then Judy, one of the nurses, came in and took a look at Hank and started laughing. "Hank, why do you have all that stuff in your ears and in your nose?"

"There's more," I told her, as she started adjusting the IV of the man in the next bed, who seemed to be sleeping. "Under the gown."

Judy looked at Hank and raised her eyebrows.

"Hank says that he needs more morphine."

Judy sighed. "Hank, this is the third time in the last hour that you've asked. You aren't due until three."

"What time is it?"

"It's quarter after two."

"Can I have it early?" Hank looked at me. "I really need some more."

"Hank," I said, "we increased your dose this morning. I think we ought to see if it is going to work."

"But I need some more. There was blood from my penis."

"Is that painful now?"

"Yes."

"When was the last time that you had bleeding or drops of blood from your penis?"

"I don't know, maybe yesterday." As Hank spoke his eyelids began to droop and he looked as if he might fall asleep.

"Hank?"

"Yeah?" He opened his eyes.

"Hank, are you falling asleep?"

"Come on, Hank," said Judy. "Get your feet up and get in bed. You're always doing this; you want more pain medication but you're falling asleep from it."

"Have you seen any blood from his penis?" I asked her.

"No. When he came up from the ER two days ago the report said that there had been some blood when the Foley was pulled, but since then he's been using the bathroom and we haven't seen any."

"What about his ears?"

Judy looked at Hank again. "Why do you have that stuff in your ears, Hank?"

Hank appeared to be struggling to open his eyes. "They were itching," he said.

Hank seemed to be dozing.

"I'll come back a little later to see you, Hank."

"I need some more morphine," I heard him say from his bed.

"We'll talk about it in a little while." I walked out of the room with Judy and went with her to the medication record that the nurses keep with all the doses of medications given to the patients. Two days ago Hank had come to the emergency room with back pain, a fever, and malodorous urine. Diagnosed with a kidney infection, he'd required hospital admission and a few days of antibiotics. He received pain medication every four hours. The kidney infection did not arise from HIV. Hank's HIV came from a history of injection drug use. As an outpatient he participated in a methadone program, taking methadone every day to curb his body's craving for heroin. Despite the program, he continued to use other drugs and had not entirely quit heroin, either.

Judy went over Hank's pain medication dosing schedule with me. In addition to the dose every four hours, he was allowed a smaller dose of morphine every two hours if he asked for it. The nursing notes indicated that he did ask for it and had been receiving it.

"He just asks for morphine all of the time. Half the time when he asks for the p.r.n.," the extra dose, "by the time I get in there to give it to him, he's asleep. The house staff upped his dose again this morning, more to get him off their backs."

I asked Judy, "Does he ever seem to you to be in pain?"

"When we do his pain assessment he says it's ten. But, no."

"Not to me, either."

"Susan, he'll drive us nuts if you decrease his doses."

"I know this is a problem. I wish they'd called me before they increased his meds. We're going to need to detox the guy. He's clearly narcotized by all the morphine he's getting and I don't know that we are treating any pain at all. He's got a very mild pyelo," I said, "but the CT scan and the sonogram were both negative. His urine from yesterday was fine."

Perhaps somewhere in Hank's drug-addled brain he thought that his penis-wrapped attire would procure more morphine. Hank asked everyone for more morphine, even the lunch ladies delivering the trays; even the janitor with the mop who came to his room in the afternoon. He occasionally wandered out into the hall and asked a visitor or any person in a white coat who passed. I'd see him at times sound asleep in his bed on morning rounds and barely awake, barely opening his eyes, he'd ask for morphine.

I paged the resident and together we made a plan to reduce the quantity and frequency of his morphine over the next few days and not to change anything without letting each other know. We kept him on his outpatient dose of methadone as well. Without it he risked going into serious withdrawal.

Despite a lot of research and literature in the field, the world of drug and alcohol addiction remains big and sometimes murky. Many of my patients have been involved with drugs over the years, and drug use often directly caused their HIV infection, from sharing needles with other HIV-infected drug users. Drug and alcohol use could also lead to poor judgment. Patients might transmit HIV through uninhibited sexual behaviors.

Of course we learned about drugs and alcohol in medical school. We studied the different chemical compounds and how they worked when ingested or injected or inhaled. We learned about toxic substances and overdoses and how to treat or manage the ill effects of chemicals. The HIV epidemic introduced a new way for drug use to be potentially lethal.

We weren't, however, taught how to deal with drug addicts. "Addiction Medicine" hadn't been born so we learned about addiction medicine through our experiences as we traveled through medical school and residency and into our roles as physicians. Psychiatrists always had a lot more training and experience with drug-using or drug-addicted patients.

Beyond HIV, drug use could lead to a variety of medical complications, not the least of which, of course, was an overdose. More often, however, the hospitalized patients had a different problem: an infection related to dirty syringes, a heart attack or stroke, or for CSS patients an opportunistic infection. In all these cases the doctors had to deal with the patient's drug use in addition to their medical issues. More than with other drugs, heroin-addicted patients suffered dramatically if they went into withdrawal. We tried to avoid this by giving them methadone, but methadone came with its own problems and many patients refused it, insisting on a different narcotic.

Methadone works on specific pain receptors in the brain and can be very helpful in eliminating the physical craving that addicts experience when deprived of heroin. Detractors say its use just trades one addiction for another. Methadone maintenance involves taking methadone every day to substitute for taking heroin. Motivated patients in recovery can often negotiate with their methadone clinic to pick up their methadone once a week instead of every day. Sometimes patients gradually decrease their methadone dose over many months and are able to be drug-free. This doesn't occur that often. More frequently, patients get themselves off methadone too fast and turn to heroin again.

We learned the expression "drug-seeking behavior" and experienced firsthand how manipulative, entitled, and demanding drug-seeking patients could be. Some whined, others begged; some used charm and others tried personal insults to get what they wanted. Patients who constantly demanded more pain medication could be very draining for the already busy and harried nurses and residents.

I learned a lot about drug use from my patients and I admired the ones who'd been able to leave drugs behind. I had several patients for whom an AIDS diagnosis served as their wake-up call. One man named Brian had arms totally covered with little round scars from where he'd injected drugs under his skin after his veins became too scarred up. He'd begun using drugs at age eleven. Brian got an HIV test when he developed fungus in his mouth. The diagnosis shocked him. He suddenly had the feeling that he was going to die. All the years of drugs had never caused him to look at himself or his life and how he was living it. The positive HIV test "saved" him; he completely stopped using drugs and didn't even go into a methadone program. He went back to school for his high school diploma, then took drug-counseling training courses. He got a job and worked hard, proving himself to be reliable and appreciated. When I saw him in the office he never dwelled on his past; but if I asked about it he'd tell me stories of friends who were dead or family members who had lost their lives in their struggles with drugs. He'd say, "Without

AIDS, who knows where I'd be now. I could be dead by now." His smile filled
the room. "AIDS is the best thing to ever happen to me!"

I wished I had more patients like Brian. For many of my patients drugs
existed as an underlying theme of much of their lives, a theme that surrounded them and the people they loved. I spent time in my office hours
encouraging active drug users to get into programs or go to meetings to beat
their drug habit or their alcoholism. Some people had no interest in this conversation, no glimmer of motivation to stop. My words sounded empty and
hollow even to me at these times, my intrusion unwelcome and my words dis-
regarded. I didn't know where to go with my counseling when a patient didn't
even acknowledge the drug use, or had no intention of stopping. Occasionally
a patient came to the office high or drunk. Nothing particularly helpful came
out of these unproductive visits. Sometimes I just didn't have the energy to
talk about it. After reviewing Hank's morphine schedule, I let the resident
and Judy know that we'd be trying to taper the medication slowly in the days
ahead.


Maggie and Suzette stood in the hall next to the nurses' station. Suzette
had her hand on Maggie's shoulder. "Tom-Tom," she mouthed at me as I
approached. Maggie looked up at me and tried to smile, her face blotchy with
tears.

"Oh, Maggie." I put my hand on her arm, tears coming to my eyes. Poor
Maggie. "How's Rodney?" I asked.

"He was admitted this morning. His kidneys are failing."

"Oh." I could only shake my head. "I'm so sorry." It felt as if the recent
support group had taken place a hundred years ago and yet the inevitable was
now reality. Maggie's "Tom-Tom" dead and his lover in the hospital. Maggie
struggled to gain her composure. We all were on our way down the hall to the
eleven a.m. inpatient rounds. I reached out and gave Maggie a hug.


Once a week, on Fridays, we held multidisciplinary rounds in the solarium
to review the inpatients on our floor in the hospital. We sat in the big,
bright room and discussed every hospitalized patient who carried a diagnosis of HIV. Even patients on surgical or obstetrical services were presented,
because we were invariably called upon to see them. Rarely, an HIV patient
received care from one of the hospital's private attending physicians, but the

CSS social worker visited these patients often as well. Any CSS staff member involved with a patient in the hospital came to Friday rounds, including the nurses on our inpatient floor, as well as Dr. Jacobs and Gerald, our administrator. In contrast to the outpatient rounds we held each day after clinic on the twenty-fourth floor, Friday rounds solely addressed hospitalized patients and allowed the inpatient nurses to participate and hear from the doctors, social workers, psychiatrists, nutritionist and other service providers all in one meeting.

The nurse read out the patient's name. The doctor described why the patient was in the hospital and what the plans were for his or her care. The nurse summarized the patient's current progress, including whether there were tests scheduled and any issues such as ongoing fever or inadequate pain control or difficult behavior. The psychiatrist, if involved, spoke next, and then the social worker, the nutritionist, the physical therapist, and the chaplain. We tried to be brief, as these rounds usually covered between twenty and forty-five patients. If a patient's hospitalization had been lengthy or there were complicated issues to discuss, it could take a while to get through everyone on the list.

Friday rounds took a more formal approach than our usual daily clinic rounds upstairs. Perhaps it was Dr. Jacobs's presence or the participation of the inpatient floor nurses that gave these rounds added weight. It may have simply been that the inpatients were so sick. Our patients came into the hospital for conditions that we often could not treat and sometimes could not even diagnose. Many were dying, not on this admission but perhaps on the next. A patient might go home for a time but would be back too soon. Or be so ill that he or she could no longer go home and we needed to arrange for placement in a nursing home. I never got used to the idea of discharging a thirty-year-old man to a nursing home. Or a woman with three young children at home needing to make arrangements with a relative or friend for the care of the children because she, the mother, could no longer do it herself and likely would never be able to. The gravity of what we dealt with in the hospital found focus in Friday rounds.

And yet rounds were rarely gloomy. We relied on one another and drew strength from our mutual caring and commitment. We shared an enormous capacity for humor, and as we discussed situations both tragic and macabre, the sense that we were participating in something bigger than ourselves prevailed. We used humor to let off steam and to temper the tragedy. It also kept us from taking ourselves too seriously. On Fridays we had snacks during rounds. Dr. Jacobs tended to hoard the potato chips and Stan would occasionally reprimand him: "Quit hogging the chips."

Dr. Jacobs's quiet, dry wit often set the tone. Stan once presented a patient who'd had a long and difficult course and who seemed to be deteriorating despite what sounded like nearly heroic efforts on Stan's part. As Stan stopped speaking there'd been a short silence in the room, broken by Dr. Jacobs saying, "Well, if the poor man had had a real doctor he wouldn't be in this mess." Stan rolled his eyes and shook his head.

Later in the same rounds the nurse gave the name of a patient being treated by Dr. Jacobs, who reviewed the challenging, discouraging case. At the end Stan asked, "Who is this poor man's doctor?" Dr. Jacobs joined in our laughter. These comments did not diminish the seriousness or difficulty, but in their roundabout way they acknowledged our recognition of one another. Lifting the burden a bit was part of our team approach. As with the regular clinic rounds, inpatient rounds offered an opportunity to get advice or support, or let off steam or frustration. I looked forward to presenting Hank, to hearing if anyone had any ideas on how to handle him.

On this Friday the list held thirty-three patients. We went through them one by one. The impressive array of medical issues bore witness to the many ways in which the human body became vulnerable when a certain aspect of the immune system didn't function. Opportunistic infections were the hallmark, but we saw AIDS take its toll on virtually every organ in the body. Heart, lungs, kidneys, liver, brain, skin—all and more could potentially manifest the effects of the virus. While on one level intellectually fascinating, the course of the disease could also be scary and horrible. A lot of the rules of medicine went out the window with patients who had multiple problems all at once, or went from stable to critically ill in a matter of hours. We learned to be vigilant and to listen. Often the labs or the CT scans or the X-rays would not tell us why a patient had a given complaint or symptom. We learned to recognize the patterns and make decisions on care based on previous trends and experience. It definitely felt at times more like art than science.

"Hank D.," said the nurse.

A couple of the nurses groaned and I saw some knowing smiles around the room.

I cleared my throat and gave my spiel. "Hank is my patient, a forty-two-year-old former and current heroin user who is here with pyelonephritis improving on antibiotics. He has been afebrile for two days so I would like to discharge him soon but I'm having difficulty weaning his narcotics.

His T cell count is three hundred and sixty, and aside from the morphine and antibiotics he's on no other medication."

Judy, Hank's nurse, with whom I'd spoken earlier, sighed before she began. "Hank is afebrile today and his vital signs are stable. He remains on IV antibiotics and he is up and about in his room. He does not seem to be in pain but he asks for morphine about every hour and is driving the nurses and the house staff crazy." Judy and I looked at each other and shrugged our shoulders.

Dr. Berry spoke next. "Hank has been in the downtown methadone program for about two years but continues to use intermittently. He has a narcissistic personality disorder with borderline features and is seeming to take advantage of being in the hospital to get as high as he can from the morphine that he gets for pain."

"He's really tough," I said. "The pyelo shouldn't be a cause of pain for him at this point. It seems that half the time when he asks for morphine he's barely awake."

Dr. Berry nodded. "I know. I'll talk to him after rounds. I'll put a note in the chart for the house staff to help them manage it. I think it can be tapered pretty quickly. We have to be firm with him."

Briana was Hank's social worker. She spoke next. "Well, Hank usually asks me for morphine, too." There was a chuckle around the room. "He's a forty-two-year-old heterosexual male who was diagnosed with HIV in 1989. His risk factor is injection drug use. He lives in supportive housing downtown and has Medicaid and food stamps. We will help him get transportation when he is discharged. I told him he'd have to ask the doctors for the morphine."

Next was Miranda, our nutritionist. "Me too," she said. "Morphine. I find that he has a good appetite and although he is thin he reports always being a skinny kid and getting teased for this when he was little. I have him in for extra portions and liquid supplements."

"And morphine?" Dr. Jacobs asked.

"Actually I wondered if anyone saw him this morning when he was in the bathroom," said Miranda.

"Oh yes," said Judy and I at the same time.

Miranda blushed. "Well, I didn't know what to say. What was all that tissue paper doing in his ears? Or around his . . . ?" She paused and made a vague, embarrassed gesture toward her lap. "I mean he was pretty naked."

"Wait a minute," said Stan. "Hank wrapped his Johnson in toilet paper? And had nothing else on?"

"Well, there was a lot of paper in his ears, too."

Judy snorted with laughter.

"It was quite a sight," said Miranda.

"I'm sorry I missed it," said Stan with a chuckle.

"Harriet?" This was from Gerald, keeping the rounds moving.

Sister Harriet had worked at CSS for three years. She visited all of the patients, usually starting her visit with assurances that she visited everyone as part of her job. Invariably the first time she walked into a patient's room and announced that she was the chaplain, the patient thought the worst. Sister Harriet allayed that fear and offered to pray with people if they were open to it or just to explore their spiritual ideas or feelings. Harriet had lived for many years in the Bronx and there seemed to be little that rattled her. She rattled, though. She smoked heavily and she had a constant bad cough. She always spoke last at inpatient rounds.

"Hank was born Pentecostal but is no longer practicing. He asked me for morphine too, but instead I suggested a prayer."

"I'm sure that was very satisfying for him," said Dr. Jacobs.

"Well, he fell asleep before I started."

"Well, Harriet, I hope that you weren't insulted."

"I hope God wasn't insulted," said Stan.

"No," said Sister Harriet. "I think God was OK about it."

"Maybe Hank could get God to give him some more morphine," Dr. Jacobs suggested. "Harriet, can you help him with that?"

"Oh."

"Did you happen to see Hank this morning in his outfit?"

"No, I missed that, fortunately."

"Thank God."

I was amazed at first at this banter that went on in rounds. It seemed so irreverent. It *was* so irreverent. But as we moved on to the next patient, I felt my own stress and frustration with Hank ease up. I had company, and my colleagues had cases just as hard or just as discouraging. The anxiety and worry spread out and dissipated in the room. I asked Dr. Jacobs to please pass the chips.

After we finished I went back to see Yolanda again. I'd looked in on her quickly that morning so I could present her at inpatient rounds, but my visit had been too rushed. I wanted to go back and talk to her and examine her. Yolanda had a recurrent herpes infection. Her third episode in the last six months, this outbreak had come on with snarling aggression and intensity. Horrible to look at, excruciating to experience, Yolanda's entire genital area was an open sore. She needed to be hospitalized because she couldn't walk and she couldn't sit. She lay silently in her bed day after day. Already two weeks had passed. The nurses whispered at the medication station that they'd never seen anything so gruesome or painful. I had to make a conscious effort not to cringe at the site of her wound when I examined her.

A tough broad, a lesbian from the South Bronx, Yolanda spoke with a deep voice and dressed in denim and leather. She had a crew cut and multiple piercings in her ears. A black tattoo on her left arm said *Milagros* in script. She kept to herself and rarely complained, but Yolanda did not hesitate to swear at the nurses when she was irritated or when she didn't want to do what they asked her to do. All movement was painful; even something as simple as changing her bedsheets became an ordeal and her foul language could be heard up and down the halls.

Beneath Yolanda's tough attitude I sensed a lonely vulnerability about her. She rarely looked me in the eye and she answered my questions in brief sentences without elaboration. I never saw a visitor in her room or a card or flower on her bedside table. One of our social workers, Mikla, had known Yolanda from a previous support agency and they had a good rapport. Mikla told me that Yolanda's girlfriend, not someone named Milagros, was also HIV-positive. The girlfriend had recently started sleeping with Yolanda's brother.

Herpes outbreaks usually resolve on their own within a week or so, but in our patients the lesions could be much more destructive and could last many weeks. Acyclovir, the only treatment we had for herpes, did not always work. We did what we could to support people with intravenous fluids and antivirals, but we had to be patient and wait. We waited for Yolanda's infection to run its course. Her condition improved slightly every day but it was slow going. She didn't like to ask for the powerful medication that eased the pain but knocked her out. She lay there and waited.

Everyone who went into Yolanda's room was required to wear a mask, hair covering, a clean gown, and gloves. This protected her, we hoped, against outside germs causing an infection on top of the open wound. For me, it felt like putting on layers of distance from Yolanda. I didn't like the mask, especially. I didn't like to have my face hidden from her. She could be difficult and her language could be intimidating but I wanted to reach her somehow and the mask just made it harder.

Yolanda rested quietly in her bed; I'd rarely even seen her watch television. She wore a hospital gown over a dark blue T-shirt. Acyclovir dripped into her arm through her IV but it didn't seem to be doing a lot of good. I knocked and stepped into her room. Yolanda lay on her back with her face turned away from the door. The brightness outside the window highlighted her pallor and the shadows under her eyes.

"Hi," she said desultorily, looking over at me.

"Hi, Yolanda. How are you today?"

"Same as fucking ever," she said looking back toward the window.

"Miserable?"

She didn't answer.

"Yolanda, can I take a look at your wound? The nurse said she's coming in a few minutes to help you wash. I'd like to see if there's any change there."

Without looking at me Yolanda shifted in her bed and I pulled back her sheet to examine the area between her legs. She lay on a disposable bed cover. Though not deep, her wound dripped constantly and the lesions themselves had spread beyond her genital area down her thighs. The red and oozing confluence covered her entire labia and half of her buttocks. No healthy tissue remained. I knew I was seeing something that few people had ever seen. A routine herpes outbreak never caused such a ghastly wound. HIV had wrecked her body's capacity to fight back. The herpes was taking full advantage of Yolanda's compromised immunity. But while the center area remained very angry and red, I felt relieved to see that the edges had dried a little and bore the telltale pink color of healing tissue.

"Yolanda, I see a little bit of healing here. That's great. Are you OK though? Are you getting enough pain medication?"

"I hate that stuff. I feel like a zombie."

"I know you don't ask for it often but I don't want you to be having too much pain. This is what the medicine is for."

"My sister died of an overdose. I don't want that shit."

Her comment came as a surprise. This was more than she'd ever said to me. As I pulled the sheet back up gently over her legs to her waist, I asked her, "When did your sister die?"

"She died when I was twenty-eight. She was thirty-three." Yolanda didn't look at me; she continued to stare out the window.

"I'm sorry. That must have been very hard for you." I heard the words as they came out and immediately felt embarrassed to be saying something that sounded so clichéd, so hollow.

"We used to shoot up together."

"Oh." I didn't know what to say to her. What could that possibly have been like? Yolanda hadn't done any drugs in five years. I wondered if her sister's death had been what prompted her to stop using. "Is that how you got infected?"

"Yeah." She paused. "Who knows? What the fuck?"

Indeed. She was right. "Yeah." It was all I could think of to say.

"You don't know. This sucks." She glanced at me with dark, angry eyes.

I searched around for something to say to her. We came from different worlds; I couldn't know her pain, her life, and I wasn't pretending to. Her pain filled the room and I felt ineffective and sad at my inability to help her medically or connect with her emotionally. All I could do was be here with her and offer her some support, some company in this grim and lonely time. "Yolanda, you're getting a little better. I know you're discouraged. It's horrible what you're dealing with. I do see some improvement though. Does your family come? Do you want me to call them?" Mikla had told me there were parents somewhere, in the Bronx perhaps.

She didn't look at me. "No," she said softly.

"I'm sorry."

"It doesn't matter."

I stood there for a moment. It was as if there was a big barbed wire fence between us. Neither of us had put up the fence but there it was; I couldn't get to her. Yolanda's pain and loneliness stuffed the space between us.

Unexpectedly, she turned on her side toward me and her fingers reached out and traced the numbers on the phone sitting on the bedside stand. We both watched the circular motion of her hand on the phone. "Dr. Ball, why did I get this?"

I looked at her face, her brown eyes ringed with purple shadows. My throat caught; I couldn't help at all. I was this woman's doctor but I could not come close to easing her suffering. Her sister was dead, her girlfriend and brother had betrayed her, and her body was torn by constant pain from a wound that dripped and hurt and wouldn't heal. Her parents lived in their own world off somewhere and they didn't visit her.

"Oh, I wish I knew. Yolanda, I wish I had an answer that would make any sense." I watched her fingers and hoped that she wasn't looking at me. A large tear slid down my nose. I blotted at it with the mask that covered half my face. For a long time neither of us said anything. Out in the hall someone's name was paged overhead. Yolanda's fingers stopped tracing and she lay there quietly, staring at the phone, and I wondered if anyone ever called her. What did she think about? Where did she go?

We both looked up as the nurse came into the room and fiddled with the intravenous bags. I realized I should get back up to my office. I stepped away from Yolanda's bed. The nurse looked at us, me standing with tears on my face and Yolanda silent as always. "I'll be back in just a moment with your meds, Yolanda," she said and discreetly left the room.

I stood for a moment longer. "Yolanda, I know this is really hard. I wish I could tell you how you got this and I wish I could tell you that everything is fine. You've been very brave and patient. We're doing the best that we can and your wound does look better. I'll see you tomorrow. I hope you get some rest." As I walked out she continued to lie there, again tracing the phone numbers with her fingers.

Yolanda got here because of AIDS but she got AIDS because of drugs, as did Hank, Brian, and so many other patients in my care. Hank wanted more narcotics but Yolanda and Brian both rejected their addiction to drugs. Good drugs and bad drugs, I thought. I wished I had the former, to be able to treat this virus and make a difference for my patients. Would we ever find something that worked? Yolanda's suffering etched itself into my brain. As I walked down the hall, my efforts at finding words of encouragement for Yolanda echoed meagerly in my ears. I could go to the nurses' station and write an order for intravenous medications which were proving unhelpful. I wrote one for narcotics which she declined to accept. What Yolanda really needed was a friend. I couldn't write an order for a friend. Time, good nursing care, compassion, all might help a little, but Yolanda's suffering came from more than her medical condition. I thought I'd speak to Sister Harriet about her. Then I smiled to myself thinking about the four-letter language barrier.

# Chapter Five

# 1994 Being Mindful of the Subtext

Two years at CSS passed quickly. By 1994 nearly 300,000 people had died from AIDS in the United States, and worldwide the estimates of those infected exceeded 10 million, yet still we lacked any significant treatments for HIV. A study of a possible vaccine to prevent HIV transmission had ended in complete failure. At the annual International Conference on HIV/AIDS in Berlin, we heard the results of a study that only confirmed what our clinical practices had taught us about AZT: it couldn't stop the virus and it had barely any effect on slowing the progression of the disease. It did, however, reduce the transmission of HIV from an infected mother to her unborn child.

Patients clamored for something, anything to halt the virus or bolster their failing immune systems. Alternative therapies flared and died like shooting stars as patients traveled across the world for potions and cures that had no medical reliability. We heard about bitter melon, Peptide T, and ozone as well as hyperthermic treatment of the blood and therapies ranging from herbs and gems to magnetic fields. I cautioned my patients against those magic options that sounded like mere quackery but I couldn't argue against the wild terror that drove people to try unproven therapies.

The lack of effective therapy had, over time, stimulated a strident activism. A real and justifiable sense that many patients with HIV were dying because of stigma prompted patients, their loved ones, and even many in the medical community to work together to voice their anger and frustration and make some changes. Congressional foot-dragging and the catatonically slow pace of new drug approval led to protests and sit-ins and people chaining themselves to the front gates of drug makers. This activism did not go unheard, particularly in the area of new drug development, and increasing numbers of medications were "fast-tracked" by regulators to get them approved while maintaining the requirements for safety.

Without effective HIV medication many of my patients died; it was too depressing to keep track of exactly how many. I just knew the number increased every month. Rumors of new drugs abounded, but for many patients such options would not arrive fast enough. I saw new patients steadily, either in my office or in the hospital. I scheduled visits every two or three months for my stable outpatients.

With so many of my people sick, I spent a lot of time making rounds in the hospital. Sometimes, if I had a gap in my schedule, I'd run down to the hospital floor or the emergency room in the middle of my office hours to see a patient. "Run down" is an exaggeration, as the two old elevators stopped on nearly every floor from twenty-four down. I also conferred with the floor nurses or the residents by phone if there were decisions to be made or test results to discuss.

While the stable clinic patients may not have been on the verge of death, many came to their appointments with pressing non-medical issues. Some days the parade of their insolvable social or psychiatric problems wore me down and I greatly appreciated the help provided by my colleagues in those disciplines. I frequently saw patients whose troubles had less to do with their HIV infection than with damaged childhoods, poverty, lack of family support, bad decisions, or unending entitlement. Of course adding HIV to this mix didn't help.

Olive always scheduled her appointments as my first patient of the day. I got to the office some mornings and stifled a little groan when I saw her chart on my door. It meant she was here, in the waiting room, waiting for me. It meant my day would start with a patient who drove me nuts. Olive was a bottomless pit of medical complaints. I fell into that pit every time I saw her. I could hear my own voice echoing for miles down in the depths.

Olive's husband hadn't told her that he injected heroin between his toes and sometimes had anal sex with other men. By the time he was diagnosed—he later died from PCP—he and Olive had a four-year-old son. Then Olive found out that she was infected. Their son did not have the infection.

Olive had been coming to CSS since it first opened and I became her doctor when I took over from my predecessor. Despite several years of HIV infection her T cell count hadn't declined very much and she'd had no HIV-related illnesses. Before I met her for the first time I read through the CSS clinic notes, which contained a long list of problems and medications. Then, as I talked to her, I tried to separate out the major issues from the minor ones. Olive requested renewals on a number of the listed medications, and I pulled out my pad and wrote what seemed like a dozen or more prescriptions, mostly for over-the-counter medications that would be paid for by her insurance if I wrote a prescription. When she asked for "my antibiotics" I stopped and looked up at her.

"What are the antibiotics for?"

"It's for when I need them."

"Well, you know, I'm not sure that's a good idea."

"Well, Dr. Yankaur did it and I know my body. I know when I need antibiotics."

At this moment I knew that things were heading downhill.

"Olive, I would prefer it if you would call me if you are feeling—"

She interrupted. "I know my body, Dr. Ball, it's my body and I know when I need to take antibiotics. Dr. Yankaur always gave them to me and if I have some left over I take them when I need them the next time."

I felt the downhill slide pick up speed. Stopping and starting antibiotics leads to antibiotic-resistant bacteria. It is a big problem in medicine and I often spent time talking to patients about the correct use of antibiotic prescriptions. "There's a problem if you have leftover antibiotics."

"I don't know why you're giving me a hard time about this. Dr. Yankaur never did and I've been coming here for three years."

"Olive, listen, we're just getting to know each other and there's a lot that you haven't told me about. I'd like to look at the hospital records; all I have here is Dr. Yankaur's notes from your visits up here, not the visits of the other doctors you've mentioned. I'm not comfortable right now with giving you medicine just to have on hand. We can talk about it again but for today I'm just going to give you these other prescriptions."

She didn't argue any further but she clearly wasn't happy with me. She complained to the social worker and to the administrator that I wasn't giving her "her" medicine. That first meeting left me with an unsettled feeling as well. I regretted that we were off to a bad start but I didn't intend to give patients medications that they didn't need. Nor did I want to be treated like a waitress, serving up a menu of any medication the patient ordered.

Shortly after our first visit I got a chance to look at her old records. Three thick charts full of visits to all kinds of doctors, lab results from hundreds and hundreds of blood tests, and X-rays and CT scans of every conceivable part of her body. Olive had what we call a somatiform disorder. She would develop a certain complaint and present it to her doctor, who found nothing wrong on exam but ordered some kind of test just to be sure. The complaint would persist despite normal test results, so more involved tests would be done. Olive would be sent to a specialist—a pulmonologist, for example, or an ear, nose, and throat doctor. Sometimes medications were ordered to alleviate Olive's symptoms but they would not help. Even more invasive tests, biopsies, and elaborate scans would follow. Twice she'd had surgery to evaluate a complaint of pelvic pain. The surgery didn't reveal anything wrong. Biopsies came back normal. When the surgery was over and the postoperative course had allowed the incision to heal, Olive gradually got back on her feet and resumed her daily life.

Then there would be a new problem.

Not all complaints led to surgery. Many would stop at the specialty clinics and elaborate tests with normal results. Olive had had so many CT scans and X-rays and ultrasounds that the radiology department knew her by name. The three thick charts revealed dozens of unsuccessful pursuits of ultimately evanescent complaints.

She'd had headaches and tingling feet, palpitations and muscle spasms, seizures, diarrhea, fainting, itching, eye pain, stomach pain, asthma, bursitis, arthritis, conjunctivitis, whateveritis. I ordered tests and more tests. Initially, as her doctor, I tried to assess and treat each problem; I tried to make her better. I sent Olive to specialists and when she came back and said the specialist suggested a different test, I ordered that one, too. I became frustrated with her chronic complaints, the normal test results, and the seemingly ineffective attempts at treatment. I found myself referring her to specialists sooner rather than later. Once I sent her to the surgery clinic as soon as she mentioned that she had abdominal pain. I did not order a single test. The resident in the surgery clinic called to yell at me. He wanted a reason to operate; he didn't want some HIV-infected lady with abdominal pain and no workup. I laughed when I hung up the phone. My transparent attempt to get someone else to do my job was pretty pathetic.

Sometimes I found her thick medical charts insulting; there were so many patients dying from HIV. Here was this woman whose HIV was not a problem in the least, but who was costing tremendous amounts of time and resources. It took me a while to see how much I was contributing to the problem with Olive. Her suffering was real, but its cause was not something that tests or biopsies or pain pills would alleviate.

She had been abused as a child and endured tremendous physical and psychological trauma. She unconsciously took refuge in the sick role, and I didn't really start taking care of her until I stopped responding to her complaints with tests or medications. Instead I sent her to see Dr. Prin, one of our two psychiatrists. At my suggestion that she see a "shrink," Olive berated me for not taking her seriously. But after a few visits with her, Dr. Prin got Olive to say that she took comfort in being sick. This declaration didn't cure her. Her refuge in the sick role was unconscious, and saying it out loud didn't suddenly make her a different person. In fact, the person who probably benefited the most from Olive's seeing Dr. Prin was me. While she still frustrated me, I felt more compassion for her need for attention. Olive had no epiphany, but it seemed like progress to have some understanding on her part that being sick was a way to escape from reality.

One thing that always seemed miraculously to cure Olive was a trip. She and her boyfriend went on vacation two or three times a year. They went on cruises or tours. They went to Alaska and Hawaii and the Caribbean islands. They went to California and Spain and New Orleans. We assumed that her boyfriend paid for these holidays as Olive had no income of her own. One day Olive would be in my office complaining of horrible, crippling dizzy spells and two weeks later would come in with pictures of her smiling at the midnight buffet during her week spent on a cruise ship off Mexico. No, she hadn't been dizzy at all during the trip. I told her I wished I could write her a prescription for a cruise whenever she came in with a new problem. I wasn't kidding.

One day, more than a year into my job, Olive wanted a letter to excuse her from jury duty.

"Dr. Ball, you know I can't sit there for jury duty."

"Have you ever gone for jury duty?"

"No, I've always gotten a doctor's letter. Doctors don't think I should be on the jury, it's too stressful for me."

"Doctors have always written letters for you?"

"My doctors don't want me on jury duty."

"But do you want to be on it?"

"No."

"Is there something that is wrong that you can't do it?"

"Dr. Ball, I have asthma, I have headaches, I have HIV. I can't be there with all those people. My doctors have said that it's not good for me."

Patients often asked for jury duty excuse letters and I've written a lot of them. Some patients clearly needed them and could not perform their jury duty even if they wanted to. But there were patients for whom the question of whether they were sick or not was rarely part of the equation; they simply didn't want to go down to the courthouse to do all that waiting around. For a moment I debated trying to discuss whether or not Olive could actually perform jury duty. It was a short debate. Olive had no intention of serving on a jury and she was not asking for a letter; she was waiting for the letter that there was no question I would write. If Olive could go on a cruise, why couldn't she be on a jury? I hated feeling manipulated. I had this image in my head of two schoolgirls on the playground arguing over whose turn it was to use the slide. I bit my lip and wrote her letter for her. I needed to have some kind of give-and-take with her and I needed to pick the battles that I would wage. This was not one of them. Although I didn't say anything that wasn't true, I didn't mention her recent cruise. Olive didn't ask me again about the CT scan that another doctor had suggested to investigate her runny nose. This, I suppose, was our trade-off for the day.

Luz came in for a routine appointment. I hadn't heard from her in weeks. When I went out to the waiting room to call her, I noticed an enormous change from the last time I'd seen her. She needed to have the fluid from her belly removed again.

"Wow, Luz, you are really big," I said as she walked toward me.

"I know, just in the last few days it has gotten so much worse."

"Come on into the office."

If you glanced at her, you'd think that Luz had a hugely pregnant belly. But her arms and legs were thin and her face, too, was thin. Her liver had failed and could no longer process and distribute her body's nutrients and fluids. She was starving, while water—known as ascites—collected in the abdomen because the liver couldn't function. Luz's swollen and taut belly must have been carrying an extra three gallons or more.

"This all happened in the last few days?"

"Well, it's been slowly getting bigger and I was going to call you but it wasn't hurting or anything and I didn't want to bother you. I knew I had my appointment coming."

"Did you miss your last appointment?"

"I couldn't get here. It was raining and Toby was home with the flu."

"Oh, I was thinking that I hadn't seen you since you went home from the hospital. When was that?"

"It was about two months ago."

"Did the swelling start right after you went home?"

"It did a little. The medicine seemed to make it go slower and I was being very careful about having my feet up. That seemed to help for a while. But then, I don't know, the kids were out of school for a few days and things just got worse."

"You look pretty miserable. Have you weighed yourself?"

"Well, I haven't been eating much. And my breath is short."

"What was your regular weight before all of this started? You were one fifty-five in June of last year; does that sound about right?"

"Yeah, I'm usually about a hundred and fifty-five, but then I went down to a hundred and forty."

"And now you're one seventy-five."

"I am?"

"Yes. That's what the nurse wrote down. And it looks like it's all in your belly because your face looks thin to me. Let's try to get some of this fluid off to at least make you a little more comfortable."

Luz's liver failure came from hepatitis C. Long associated with blood transfusions, this illness frequently occurred in patients who used injection drugs like heroin and cocaine. Hepatitis C is also transmitted through sexual contact. The hepatitis C virus took a while to identify. We had only recently stopped calling the illness non-A, non-B hepatitis.

Hepatitis A is usually a mild infection that resolves in all patients. While more serious, in 90 percent of patients hepatitis B also clears from the body spontaneously. Unfortunately, hepatitis C lingers on as a chronic infection in nearly 85 percent of those infected. A significant percentage of those with chronic hepatitis C develop liver failure over many years. These patients also have a higher risk of developing liver cancer. Screening of the blood supply has dramatically reduced the risk of transfusion-associated hepatitis C. Nonetheless, liver failure from chronic hepatitis C is the number-one cause of liver transplants in the United States.

Luz acquired her hepatitis C and her HIV from injection drug use before she stopped using ten years ago. Her T cell count remained high and she'd not had any HIV-related illness. Her liver, however, no longer worked. She'd started developing signs of cirrhosis over a year ago and the episodes of abdominal swelling were now happening with more severity and frequency. In the early 1990s liver transplant was rare enough, and HIV precluded someone from being considered for the transplant list. We didn't even think of a transplant for Luz. Her end-stage liver disease carried a dismal prognosis at this point: it was unlikely that she'd survive another year. We tried to control the swelling and fluid retention in her abdomen, but without the liver's help, ours was so much duct tape on a collapsing house.

"Do I need to be admitted?"

"Maybe not today but definitely in the next couple of days. It's a little bit up to you. I can't take the fluid off here in the office. There's too much and I need to be able to monitor your blood tests and your blood pressure in a way that I can't safely do here. I can arrange it all and hopefully you won't need to go through the emergency room. But if your breathing gets bad, you need to come here immediately."

"Can I come in tomorrow? Today I have to pick up Toby."

"OK. Do you have someone to watch the kids?"

"My sister can do it. It won't be for long, right?"

"Hopefully you'll only be in for a couple of days at the most. Will you need a ride to come here tomorrow? I forget how you get here."

"I take the subway and then the bus."

"Let me ask if Alex can come get you. If he can't, we'll get a car service for you."

Public assistance pays for an ambulette service for patients going to hospitals or clinics throughout the city, but the ambulette required three days' notice and usually picked up several other patients coming to the hospital. Alex drove the CSS van, often a quicker and easier way for our patients to get to us. The van, like so many other wonderful advantages at CSS, came from private donor money. CSS benefited from the charitable giving of many people. Several prominent New Yorkers had given to the clinic at an annual fundraiser called the Fête de Famille. The money helped provide a number of resources for us, one of which was the van and another was Alex, our full-time driver. He traveled all around the outer boroughs of the city to pick up or take home patients who could not get here on their own. Sometimes we even paid for a car service when the van wasn't available. For people like Luz, who lived far away, the van or a free ride to the clinic made all the difference when they weren't feeling well and would rather stay home than get on the subway to come to their appointment.

The elevators on the twenty-fourth floor opened directly into our large, comfortable waiting room. On the other side of the room ran a long counter behind which sat our registrars and secretaries. The door next to the counter led to the hallway and all of our offices. From the door where I stood to call in my next patient I could see a large person lying down on one of the big couches near the elevators. The person's head was covered with a dirty-looking tan raincoat. Charlene, the secretary, saw me staring in that direction and gave me a meaningful look. "That's Peaches," she said, "and she is in a foul temper." She said the word "foul" as if it had two distinct syllables, as in "fah-well."

"Ah," I said. Peaches, with her raucous laugh and itchy belly, did not have an appointment and had not been to the clinic for several months. Maybe a brief siesta on the couch would shift Peaches's "fah-well" temper to fair.

I called my next patient and Etta came in. A heavyset young woman with lovely fair skin and brown eyes, she sat across from me chewing gum, wearing a puffy light blue down vest and a magenta wool hat. She wore a touch of pink lipstick and her eyebrows were plucked to a very fine line. With her in front of me I recalled that we had had the same conversation for the last three or four appointments. Etta did not want to take any pills despite her very low T cell count. Neither of them worked very well so I didn't mind much that she refused to consider taking didanosine or AZT. What frustrated me more was that she wouldn't take anything to prevent *Pneumocystis* pneumonia. So many patients developed PCP but the prophylaxis effectively prevented it. She didn't have medication allergies and she could swallow pills if she needed to, but she simply refused. "I don't need that," she told me. I couldn't convince her. The nurses, the social worker, the nutritionist, even Sister Harriet talked to her about it. She just shook her head. "I don't want to be bothered. It's not for me." She always looked a bit annoyed in my office, and she spoke with a hint of a sneer.

Etta tested positive for HIV in 1989 while pregnant with her little son Joey. She couldn't say how she'd been infected with the virus. She didn't do drugs. She answered vaguely when I asked her if she knew whether or not Joey's father was HIV positive. "I don't know, maybe, yeah." She saw the man from time to time at the bar where she hung out but otherwise had no involvement with him. When I asked if the man knew that she had HIV she gave an indifferent shrug and response: "I don't know, it's possible, I guess."

Etta and Joey lived in a small apartment above her grandparents. Her own mother lived across the river in New Jersey and did not see her daughter or grandson very often. Etta seemed to take good care of Joey but she expressed no affection for him and often referred to him as a brat or a pain in the ass. She took him to the doctor's and got him into a special nursery school in their neighborhood. He did not have HIV. A quiet little guy, Joey poked around my desk as any four-year-old would and watched round-eyed as I listened to his mother's chest with my stethoscope.

On this visit I noted that Etta had lost weight, twenty pounds in the last four months. When I asked her if she was dieting she said no. She felt fine and did not express concern about the unintentional weight loss. Once again she refused to take any medication to protect her against *Pneumocystis*. "I feel fine." How many times had I heard that? Her previous blood work revealed a T cell count of 64. A normal count should be at least 500 or 600. She was at high risk to get PCP but somehow I could not persuade her to protect herself against it.

"Etta, what about Joey? What if you needed to be in the hospital?"

"Joey's fine. And my grandfather's a good cook. Joey eats for him better than for me."

I tried to keep my frustration under control. Was she just being stubborn? Was she stupid? Was I so much smarter or better because I wanted to protect her and keep her from getting sick? I thought I knew best. I thought my recommendations were ones she should follow. She didn't agree. Despite my exasperation, I respected Etta's independence and her self-confidence. I could give her the information, but I couldn't make her do something she didn't want to do.

Taking prophylaxis against PCP really worked; it prevented *Pneumocystis* pneumonia. Admission rates in hospitals all over the country reflected this one significant success. I had seen so many patients in the hospital with PCP. Some needed to be on breathing machines or, like John of the immaculate manicure, needed chest tubes for collapsed lungs. More patients with AIDS died of PCP in the United States than of any other opportunistic infection.

It made no sense to me that Etta refused to take prophylaxis, especially as her low T cells put her at significant risk. I blamed myself; I must not be conveying the importance of it. But the more I hammered at it, or tried to explain it differently, or insisted, the more frustrated I became. Her mind was made up and I think she barely heard me. She was like the cat in the cartoon, watching her owner talk, talk, talk and having no understanding of and less interest in what all the noise meant. Of course that made me the owner; talk, talk, talk with little or no response to my efforts. I worried about Etta and I worried about her young son. I watched her walk away from me down the hall.

I used to assume that patients who came to me wanted my help, would listen to and follow my sage doctorly advice. In fact I never deluded myself into thinking I knew all the answers, and certainly AIDS showed us we needed to be humble. Still, I thought my patients and I had similar goals: diagnosing an illness, treating symptoms and their causes, improving health. Days like today reminded me that everyone has her own agenda; my nuggets of so-called wisdom might help one patient but be only so much flotsam and jetsam for another. Luz and I wanted the same thing: she needed to feel better in order to move around and care for her son. I helped her do that. On the one hand, Olive wanted illness to excuse her from life; on the other hand, Etta behaved as if she could avoid becoming ill just by her own obliviousness. They didn't want what I offered them.

This interaction led me to think about another patient of mine, Manuel. Last year he refused to be screened for tuberculosis, a routine annual test we required of our patients as HIV puts people at higher risk to develop TB if exposed. Manuel said the test "is not on my agenda." I pointed out to him that until he'd been diagnosed, HIV had not been on his agenda either.

Manuel never smiled and rarely gave me any personal information about himself. A bit like Etta, he responded to my requests for blood tests or follow-up appointments with irritation and complaints. Thirty-two years old, Manuel had sex with men but didn't identify himself as gay. He talked about "broads" and "chicks" and bitterly referred to "the faggot" who had infected him with HIV. When I suggested he speak to Dr. Berry, that I thought he might benefit from discussing his anger with someone, he looked at me through narrowed brown eyes and said, "Oh, you think I don't know I'm angry? A fag plants a bomb in my ass—I shouldn't be angry?"

"Manuel," I said at the time, "I think you are really struggling here. I feel like the more help I can get for you the better. I'm not saying you shouldn't be angry but sometimes it can be really helpful for someone to explore where that anger comes from."

I think no one had ever spoken to him in this way. He looked down at his lap. When he looked back up at me he had tears in his eyes. "I'm sorry to give you a hard time about everything. I know you're trying to help."

He did go see Dr. Berry. At first she wondered if she could make any progress with him; he threw hostility back at her every question. But he kept going and eventually revealed a broken home and separated parents. When Dr. Berry asked him about his relationship with his father Manuel said, "If my father was on fire I wouldn't piss on him."

One Monday, Manuel came to the office unexpectedly and told me that he'd had two seizures over the weekend. His friends brought him to the local emergency room, but the friends left and after a couple of hours he felt fine, got tired of waiting, and went home. He refused when I wanted to admit him for tests but agreed to get a CT scan of his brain, which I arranged for the following morning. On Tuesday afternoon he sat across from me and listened as I told him about the ring-like lesions that lit up on the scan. The lesions had the classic appearance of cerebral toxoplasmosis, the most common of opportunistic infections involving the brain in patients with HIV. I urged him to be admitted to start treatment and make sure he didn't have any more seizures.

He shook his head. "Being in the hospital is not on my agenda."

I could not persuade him to stay in the hospital. He filled the prescriptions for the antibiotics that I gave him and called me three days later to say he'd had another seizure and been brought to the nearest hospital, where he was now an inpatient. I never saw him again.

As I went out to the waiting room to rouse Peaches from her nap on the couch, I wondered about her agenda.

"Dr. Ball, they cut my food stamps and you gotta get 'em back for me." Peaches sat heavily in the chair and immediately started scratching. She looked terrible. She wore dirty clothes and her hair stood up in bunches on her head. The rash had moved to her face and there were spots that she had scratched so hard they'd bled and scabbed over. Her fingernails were bitten down to nubs.

"Peaches, where have you been lately? I haven't seen you in months and months."

"It don't matter, Dr. Ball. I want my food stamps back."

"Did you call?"

"'Course I called. Till they disconnected my phone," she said, scowling.

"Are the boys OK?"

"They're hungry. So'm I."

"OK, I need to have the social worker talk to you and make some calls. She's the one to help with this. Have you spoken to her?"

"That woman's a pain in my ass. 'Are you smoking crack again, Peaches?'" she mimicked in a sing-song the voice of Bobsy, her social worker.

I smiled and put my head down on my hand. I knew she was right. Bobsy could be a little aggravating. "Well are you?" I asked Peaches.

"'Course I am," said Peaches. "That's how this whole fucking thing started. They just won't let me alone and I don't want to but I can't stop. I want to. I just can't. Now they cut my fucking food stamps and that fucking lady wants to tell me about detox. I don't need no detox, I need some fucking food. My kids need food!" She almost yelled this at the same time she messily wiped at her eyes and nose with the back of her hand.

"Oh Peaches," I said quietly. I gave her a box of tissues. She took them and blew her nose very loudly. She smiled at the noise.

"Fuck," she said. "Sorry, Dr. Ball."

I looked at her, discouraged. "Listen, they are going to take those boys from you again. You know that, right?"

"I'm gonna come to my appointments. I'm not doing that shit as much as before. I'm doing better. My case manager got me a home attendant. The boys don't miss school no more. I don't know why they cut my stamps and then we don't got a phone right now."

"There are some food pantries around. Have your community case manager call me and I'll have Bobsy follow up on the food stamps. I know she can bug you but she'll help, I know she will. She can give you some money for food for today. But no buying crack with it!"

"Shit. That stuff. Damn."

"I'll send you down to the lab so we can get your blood work and I'll schedule you to come back next week so that we can see the results together, then I can spend a little more time examining you. Are you OK until then?"

"I'm OK."

I walked her down the hall to the lab and Suzette. "Peaches, where have you been?" I heard her ask as I went back to my office.

This kind of day tired me out. Bad enough that HIV was so untreatable and devastating; but for some, for many, even, HIV existed as an addendum in a life that ached with need. We could barely address the HIV in those early 1990s; we had so little to offer. The need, meanwhile, was like a pit without a fence around it. I wouldn't fall in but I didn't even know how to throw a rope much less actually help anyone out.

On my way downstairs that afternoon I stood near the elevator in the waiting room. Nearby one of Stan's patients sat in a chair with his head back, resting. He looked emaciated and terrible. He had thin, brittle hair and an angry rash on his cheeks. His clothing looked three sizes too big and needed to be laundered. Just then another patient wandered by and stopped in front of the man and gazed at him for a moment. With a loud exclamation he said to Stan's patient, "Oscar! You! Look! FABULOUS!" Oscar lifted his head from the back of the chair and tiredly glanced at his admirer. With a weary little smile he puckered his lips as if to blow him a kiss. The elevator came. "Fabulous!" I heard the man say again as I stepped on and the door closed. If Oscar looked fabulous today I didn't want to imagine what he looked like when he looked sick.

# Chapter Six

# 1994 Weekend on Call

Timothy lay on a stretcher by the wall near the nurses' station. The busy emergency room bustled back and forth past him. As I approached I took in his profound emaciation, the yellow and gray skin, and the sweaty hair matted to his head. His mother stood by the stretcher and held his hand. As he noticed me, I saw that his eyes looked very tired behind his round steel-rimmed glasses.

His mother turned, following Timothy's gaze. "Oh, what a relief to see a friendly face," she said, smiling. Her face, too, looked strained and exhausted. I held out my hand and she reached out with her free hand to shake mine. I put my other hand on Timothy's shoulder. I'd met Timothy, a patient of Dr. Jacobs's, on previous weekends on call. Once when Dr. Jacobs had been unavailable, I'd seen Timothy and his mother in my office.

Now she said, "He had been doing so well on Friday night. We thought the change would do him good, you know, to get out to the country. We have a house in western Pennsylvania, near the Ohio border. Timothy was happy to go. He used to spend all his summers there. He seemed so glad and slept well when we arrived. But Saturday morning he started shivering and I knew. I just knew we should come back." She spoke in a rushed way, her voice a mixture of anxiety and fatigue.

"Oh, Mom." Timothy's voice was weak and soft. I turned toward him and saw much more than those two words. The look in his eye said she shouldn't blame herself, said he was very nearly done. It said he loved her.

"His brothers were there too. They'll be coming later. He didn't want to leave. He was having fevers and the boys were playing catch in the yard. I call them the boys. They're all grown men. We bundled him up so he could sit outside and watch." She started to cry. "He was sweating and he seemed so happy to watch them playing catch. They tossed him the ball a few times. They wanted him there with them."

"Mom."

She checked herself and took a breath. She looked back down at him and put her hand on his chest. The tenderness in her eyes as she gazed at him made my throat ache. I was worried that I might sob. But she controlled her tears and he reached up and held her hand. He had closed his eyes.

"It was clear that we had to get back. Dr. Jacobs has always recommended that we try to get here if we can. We went to the local emergency room. The hospital there is very small. They heard that he has AIDS and they got us an ambulance immediately. I think they couldn't get us out of there fast enough. And it was a long, long night but I'm glad we're here. I'm glad you're here."

"What a time you've had."

Thirty-four years old, the youngest of three sons, Timothy had a boyish smile and his damp, sandy hair usually curled off his face. I had a crush on him from the moment I met him. He had a scruffy student look that totally charmed me. I always felt that I was meeting him at the wrong time. I wished we had not been patient and doctor. In another time we would have been friends. In another time he was my classmate in medical school, he lived in my building. He shopped for smelly cheese at the store where I shopped and we laughed about it in the checkout line. He was a friend I hadn't met, but now I knew that we wouldn't. We would never get the chance to meet as friends.

Timothy's boyfriend, Andrew, had died three years ago. They'd been together for more than twelve years. In the last year or so Timothy's condition had deteriorated. His mother had moved back up from Florida to help and he was happy to have her near. Despite the anguish of the circumstances she did not want to be anywhere else. Timothy's father had died when Timothy was still in college.

"Well," I said, "I talked to the attending and he said your ambulance drivers were not helpful. Did they really just bring you in and leave without speaking to anyone?"

"They barely said a word to us for three hundred miles."

"It was good that you called me last night to let me know you were coming. I wish you didn't have to wait down here but I'm hoping a bed will open up soon."

"It's all right, Dr. Ball, everyone here has been very kind."

Timothy opened his eyes again. I looked at him and said, "Timothy, I know that you and Dr. Jacobs have discussed this before. And with your mother, too. But each time you're admitted we're supposed to ask how you feel about certain treatments that are offered in the hospital if you need them."

Timothy's mother was shaking her head and looking at the floor.

"I'm talking about whether or not you'd want to be placed on a breathing machine if you needed one. If you stopped breathing in the night, would you want to be resuscitated?"

"No," he said, very quietly.

"No, we have talked about this with Dr. Jacobs," said his mother. "After the long stay in the ICU last year, Timothy said he didn't want to go through that again."

Timothy met my eyes and shook his head. "I don't want that stuff," he said.

I nodded. "I know things have been tough these last few weeks. You've been through a lot. We're going to keep you as comfortable as we can. Your fever worries me a bit and your blood pressure is a little low. Likely there is an infection somewhere. We'll get you some fluids and antibiotics, then see what your blood tests show. I'm sure that you'll feel a bit better with some hydration. But for now no ICU, right?"

"Thank you."

"The boys are coming later?"

Timothy's mother smiled. "Yes, they're going to close up the house. Henry, the oldest, lives in Pittsburgh, so they'll stop there on their way to New York."

"That'll be good. I'm sure you'll be happy to see them. Part of the wait down here is because I want you to have your own room. It should be on our floor upstairs so you'll be able to spend the night in the room if you'd like to. The nurses are good about that. I'm on call so if there are any problems please just have me paged."

I took out my stethoscope and examined Timothy as well as I could, given the lack of privacy and the noise of the busy ER. Timothy's was not the only stretcher in the hall and everywhere there were bodies and voices. It was the typical emergency room zoo with nurses, doctors, patients, students, visitors, security guards, orderlies, and transport staff all milling about. I wished I could offer Timothy and his mother a quieter place. I looked around and found a chair for her. The thought of their long ride last night in the ambulance with an unfriendly crew bothered me. It reflected on all of us when health professionals behaved poorly. But I knew that AIDS stirred up a lot of fear and discomfort in people. I wondered if the ambulance drivers felt changed by their experience of bringing Timothy to New York. The line "after that, they were never the same" went through my mind. Death changes us. Every moment changes us.

I held Timothy's hand briefly and then shook his mother's hand again as I turned to leave. She reached out and gave me a hug. I struggled not to cry. We all knew what was coming. It was likely that Timothy wouldn't survive another month, perhaps not another week. As a doctor, I knew that my patient, this patient, was dying. Timothy knew as well. He didn't talk about it, didn't have much energy to spend thinking about it. But he knew.

His mother knew too. I could only imagine the nights and days she'd spent in the last few years thinking about it, worrying and waiting and now knowing that soon it would be true, that her son, her golden, boyish boy, her youngest, would soon be gone. I hugged her back.

I left the hospital and went out into the brilliant October day. I walked west toward Central Park and kicked up some of the fallen leaves on the sidewalk. Above me I could see the blue sky behind the branches and leaves in the trees. The air was fresh and a bit crisp with the changing season. I felt numb and dazed, a feeling I recognized from my weekends on call: leaving the hospital at four or later on a Sunday afternoon, all the rounds of Saturday and Sunday behind me. The faces and bedsides ran together, overlapped and jumbled. I watched the sky behind the leaves as I walked along. The sound of my footsteps on the sidewalk and the quiet of the street comforted me after the din of the ER. I felt myself expanding, as if I'd been holding myself in a tight, constricted pose and could now shake my arms and wiggle my fingers.

Weekends on call were one of the toughest parts of working at CSS. Stan, Maggie, and I each covered the patients for the entire weekend every four weeks or so. We hired someone to cover the other weekend. All of the patients we heard about on Friday in rounds were our responsibility, as well as the HIV patients on other services of the hospital. We consulted on new HIV-positive patients admitted to the hospital and we picked up admissions to the CSS floor. There were also phone calls from patients at home who had questions or needed prescriptions called in.

Weekend call started with the sign-out on Friday afternoon. Stan went over all his inpatients with me and let me know the things I needed to look out for, to check on, to remember. He might tell me not to see certain stable patients on other services unless I was called. He let me know if there were any patients at home with problems. Maggie gave me her sign-out too. Dr. Jacobs, Dr. Hort, and Dr. Steppin were all in private practice but they saw patients at CSS once a week on a volunteer basis. They called with their sign-outs. By Friday evening I had a list of twenty to forty-five patients to see over the weekend. I didn't have to sleep in the hospital, but often the beeper started going off promptly at five with patients or caregivers needing to talk to the doctor.

On a typical Saturday morning on call I started in the hospital before seven, doing the work rounds with the house staff. We saw and examined every patient on the service and discussed the plans for the day. These rounds could take several hours. The residents were smart, dedicated, and enthusiastic, but on the weekends there seemed to be twice as much work to do with half as many people to do it. The CSS inpatients took up an entire hospital floor, and Stan, Maggie, and I spent so much time there that we had a lot of direct contact with the residents. All of us felt that, along with the house staff, we worked together as a team, with a sense of shared responsibility and purpose. The residents appreciated the camaraderie and the support. Our involvement helped them overcome some of the fears and hesitations they might have felt in caring for patients with AIDS. Because our patients were so sick and so many of them died in the hospital, the time spent on the HIV service was considered among the most grueling in the entire training program for the medicine residents.

Rounding with the house staff on the weekends, I tried to keep us as efficient as possible and to avoid being verbose. If there were teaching points to be made I tried to be succinct and helpful. Everyone had a lot of work to do, so we focused on seeing each patient and clarifying the day's workload, knowing that any minute could bring a sudden change or a need to break away from rounds to deal with an emergency. I also felt a little insecure about how much I could teach these residents. They were an elite group. Most had been stellar medical students and came from prestigious schools. I was only a few years older than they were and I never considered myself smarter. My experiences with patients had taught me a great deal and I could convey some of that. I could dispel some of the residents' anxiety about working with AIDS patients. I could also empathize with the confusion and sadness that came from caring for a group of patients who were often young in addition to being sick and dying.

Among my colleagues in the department of medicine were some fantastic teachers. They could talk extemporaneously to students and residents about any aspect of physiology or about some detail of pathology or biochemistry. Often the clinical setting provided these colleagues an opportunity to share their knowledge. One Saturday morning I overheard one of the medicine attendings rounding with a group of residents on one of the non-HIV services, talking to them about the sodium transport in the shark rectum. I looked at the young faces as they stood around in their white coats politely listening, some of them leaning against the wall outside the patient's door, waiting for the older man to finish. My colleague was surely making an important point linking the sodium transport of the shark rectum and the care of the patient lying in the hospital bed. Sodium transport in the shark rectum may be fascinating stuff, but on a Saturday morning, with many patients to see and a reduced workforce to get everything done, I'm not sure the digression was fully appreciated. He loved teaching and the residents loved him for it. They did wish sometimes, especially on Saturdays, that he'd talk a little less.

The shark rectum lesson epitomized differences in teaching styles. Such impromptu basic science lectures contrasted with the discussions of end-of-life care or whether a patient's estranged father would come to visit his gay son in the hospital. My own teaching style focused on helping the residents learn how to care for the patients as people with real lives and real fears as much as it focused on management of opportunistic infections. Just as the physiology lectures had their place, so did the discussions of a husband in prison or a history of sexual abuse or the nearness of death. My talks had to do with putting patients' illnesses into the context of their lives as much as they had to do with patients' specific medical management. The horror and despair of AIDS made us all want to depersonalize our experiences, yet it was important to keep the residents—and ourselves—aware of the individual who lay in the bed.

By midmorning on the weekends, visitors and families were in the rooms with the patients and they often had questions for us or just wanted to chat. The later it got, the slower we would move. Sometimes rounds were interrupted by emergencies so we had to reconvene later and later. After rounds the house staff split off to go to a conference or to the ER to see their admissions. Sometimes I went back and spoke to a patient or family member by myself. Eventually, when we'd finished seeing everyone on the list, we sat down to write the notes in each patient's chart.

As I walked outside, glad the notes and rounding were done for the day, I thought about Marta and my visit with her earlier in the hospital. I had needed to speak to Marta's sister. Marta had Kaposi's sarcoma and was dying from an intestinal infection that we couldn't treat. She had no appetite and her stomach hurt all the time. Her sister or her mother often slept in the room with Marta on one of the fold-out beds that CSS provided. Kaposi's sarcoma was more commonly recognized as an AIDS-related disease of gay men, and when her initial diagnosis had been made, the pathologist had called me personally to make sure that the name Marta really indicated a female.

During the week Marta's mother had been hospitalized elsewhere with a heart attack. Tragic news, it also threw the family into chaos, as Marta's mother provided much of the caregiving for Marta's four children, who ranged in age from eleven to six. With their mother in the hospital, and now their grandmother in another hospital, the kids were frequently on their own. The nurses found them sleeping in Marta's room on two different nights. Marta's sister, Myrna, had older children of her own. The sister spent her time either in one of the two hospitals or trying to care for all of the children.

When I went into Marta's room she was watching television with the sound off. One of the children slept in her bed beside her. The other three were asleep on the pull-out bed by the window. Very little light came in around the drawn curtains.

"Hi, Marta." I leaned over the bed and spoke softly, trying not to wake the child next to her.

"Hi," she said, without looking at me. The light from the television flickered on her face.

"How are you today?"

She looked over at me. Her eyes had big gray circles under them. She looked like she could be fifty years old. "My stomach hurts," she said.

"How's the diarrhea?"

"It hasn't been bad this morning."

"Did you eat breakfast?" I saw a bowlful of soggy cereal on her tray, the bread and coffee unopened, a hardboiled egg still in its shell.

"I wasn't that hungry."

"I heard your mom is in the hospital."

"Yeah."

"You must miss her."

"Who?"

"Your mom."

"Yeah." She turned her head away from me and looked at the television. The child beside her did not move.

"Marta?"

"Yeah?"

"The kids really should not be sleeping here in the hospital."

Marta looked back at me. "It was only one night."

"Your mom or your sister, that's fine, but the kids, they aren't allowed to sleep here. Can they sleep at your sister's tonight?"

"Myrna will sleep at my house."

"So they'll sleep in their own beds?"

"Yeah."

"OK. Is Myrna coming in later?"

"Yeah, she went to see my mom and she'll be here later."

"What are your kids doing for breakfast? Did they eat something?"

"Myrna will bring McDonald's."

"Does Myrna take good care of them? Are they OK with her?"

"Yeah. Myrna helps a lot. My mom helps a lot too."

I listened to Marta's abdomen with my stethoscope and gently felt for a mass or an area of tenderness. Her belly was soft but she winced when I pressed down anywhere as I examined her.

Myrna and I had spoken about what would happen to Marta's children if Marta had to go to a nursing home, or if she were to die. Myrna would be their legal guardian should the time come. None of the children had HIV. Marta had been very resistant to signing the guardianship papers at first. In the last few months, however, she'd spent more time in the hospital than at home with her children. One day she asked her social worker to bring the papers. It was as if she suddenly knew that she wouldn't always be there to protect her children. She signed the papers and asked her sister not to talk about it anymore. No one could have predicted that the children's grandmother would not be available to help. I needed to speak to Myrna to find out how her mother was doing. Myrna was going to have a lot on her shoulders if her mother didn't easily recover from her heart attack.

"Marta, I'm on call so if you need to speak to me you can just let the nurses know and they'll page me."

"OK." The glow from the television flickered on her face. One of the children rolled over under the blanket where the others slept. Marta looked over at the three of them on the bed. Then she looked back at the television.

I went out of the room and closed the door behind me.

Usually on the weekend, when I finished my notes on our floor, I went to see all of the other HIV patients around the hospital on the other services. I saw patients in the medical ICU and the psych ward, the surgery center and the burn unit. Then I went back to our floor to work on the new admissions or finish the rounds that we had started. Some weekends, like this one, I went to the emergency room if someone was being admitted. Frequently the beeper went off with a patient at home calling with a problem or a question. I spent a lot of time talking with visiting family or friends. What was happening, what was going to happen, when will this end, when can he go home, when is her test, what does that medicine do, why isn't he talking, why isn't she eating, all the hundreds of questions to try to answer. Sometimes I sought out families to ask permission for tests or to discuss changes in the patient's status if something had happened overnight.

Despite the presence of the house staff and the nurses, and seeing all the patients and their families, despite being with people all through the long day, being on call was lonely. Without Stan or Maggie around, without bumping into a CSS social worker in the elevator or Sister Harriet in the hall, I felt like it was only me up against all this illness. During the week I'd see my own ten or twelve inpatients, but on the weekend I was responsible for *all* the patients. Only me seeing patients covered with the purple lesions of Kaposi's sarcoma, too weak to sit in a chair; patients whose lungs were connected to ventilators because they couldn't breathe well enough on their own; patients with brain tumors, unable to move; patients with eye infections slowly making them blind; patients with infections of intestines or heart or gallbladder or infections of the skin from their intravenous lines. There were patients in whose rooms no one could stay because the diarrhea was terrible and the room too foul-smelling. Some delirious patients required restraints to protect them from getting up and falling; other patients oozed blood from sores, and despite constant nursing attention their dressings or beds were always bloody. Some patients were out of their minds from infection or fever or loss of brain tissue. As the day wore on and the hours passed, every patient's illness seemed to pile up in my brain. The list went on and on.

After I left Marta, I went down the hall to see Mr. Sullivan, a man who'd been assigned to me as a new patient the day before. Mr. Sullivan had a brain cancer associated with AIDS and the cancer therapy had failed; he was now in a coma. He'd been dying at home in the care of his partner, a very dignified and thoughtful man, and as his death approached the partner found himself overwhelmed. As the patient's proxy, the partner did not wish any extreme or invasive measures to be taken to prolong Mr. Sullivan's life. He regretted having to bring him to the hospital but felt that the two had reached an understanding long ago that neither would want to be a burden to the other.

The decision had been a painful one but now Mr. Sullivan lay in a hospital bed here and his death seemed imminent.

When I went into Mr. Sullivan's room the partner was not there and I sat down in the chair between the bed and the window. I called Mr. Sullivan's name and pinched his arm lightly. He didn't move. I looked out the window for a little while and then reached over and placed my hand gently on Mr. Sullivan's knee. I could hear him breathing very slowly, sporadically. His breathing rattled. Death was coming soon, maybe in a few hours, maybe less.

I found myself thinking about Mr. Torres, with whom I used to sit from time to time when I first started at CSS, as he lay alone in an unlit room. Those times of silence, hearing the footsteps or muted voices out in the hall as I looked at his face or brushed the hair back from his brow. Now, looking at Mr. Sullivan, I wondered if I'd ever seen him before. Had I sat across from him on the subway? Jogged past him in the park? I looked up at the IV bag drooping from the pole, the liquid snaking down the clear tubing into his arm. I wondered how the nurses did it, spending their whole day here on the floor, in and out of these rooms where patients were dying. It seemed a patient died every week; sometimes more than one patient died in a day. When I started working here I wasn't very well prepared for so much terminal illness. In an abstract way I knew what to expect, but sitting here in a hospital room next to a living person as he died, I found myself thinking all kinds of things. I wondered about the life of the person lying there in the bed. I wondered about the people they loved or who loved them. Today I had an image of walking on a wooden bridge arching over a brook. I was walking with Mr. Sullivan and he would go across and I'd turn back.

Outside it was a beautiful day with a very blue sky. Mr. Sullivan's east-facing room allowed in a lot of light. Outside I could see the river and the bridge; the sun glinted off cars on the highway in the distance. Far off I could just make out the airplanes on the ground at the airport. I watched as one moved down the runway slowly and then turned and stopped. It started moving again and passed behind some buildings and trees, such a long way off from where I sat. I became conscious of the quiet in the room.

I watched as the plane, tiny and silent in the distance, rose up from the runway into the air. I kept my hand resting on the bedclothes that covered Mr. Sullivan's knee. The sky seemed very clear and the plane could be seen white against the blue as it rose higher and higher toward the west. I heard the nurse come into the room and stop next to the bed and I watched until a tall building a few blocks north hid my view of the plane.

"I think he's dead," the nurse said in a low voice.

Without looking at her, I stood up and took my stethoscope from my pocket and placed the earpieces in my ears and the round diaphragm on Mr. Sullivan's chest. I listened for a long moment to the silence there underneath the warm skin, underneath the visible ribs. The hair on his chest was straight and black with hints of gray. His skin looked very pale, like an old pillowcase. No rise and fall of faint breath, no beat or muffled sound of a heart lingering. I looked under his eyelids at his dilated pupils and staring eyes. I straightened his hospital gown a bit and pulled the sheet up to his chest as the nurse puttered with the intravenous line. We didn't speak, the nurse and I. She looked at me a bit oddly as I put my stethoscope back into my pocket. Out the window I could no longer find the airplane I had been watching. From the airport another plane rose up into the sky. I went out of the room and down the hall to the nurses' station to write the required note.

The nurses' station bustled with people and telephones and voices; it seemed noisy and blurry. The clerk had a small radio that softly played some pop music. With an awareness of being inside and outside of my body at the same time, I sensed the noise and the light and the feel of the chart in my hands. I still had the image of the wooden bridge in my mind and had a feeling of a moving stream or flow of movement passing inside me, a sense of embracing, a remove without touchstones or firm ground. I saw the plane in the blue sky and felt the soft blanket on Mr. Sullivan's knee. Almost in a daze I picked up the phone and called Mr. Sullivan's partner. The voice machine answered and the recording at the other end of the line brought me back to the nurses' station. I left a message asking Mr. Sullivan's partner to call me when he got in. He'd be here before he got the message at his home. I opened the chart and wrote a brief note at the top of the page. The rest of the page would stay blank. I closed the chart and put it back in the rack behind me. I sat for a moment more then got up and went to see the next patient.


By the time I left the hospital it was late afternoon and I felt numb. This particular sunny and crisp October day dazzled my eyes with its brightness, disorienting me in my sense of relief and the lingering stress of death and aching hearts. I felt released from a sucking hole, but I also felt guilty in my release. So thankful that I was not back there worrying or mourning at the bedside of someone I loved, or in one of those hospital beds, sick, or dying from AIDS. I thought of Timothy and his mother coming from Pennsylvania in an ambulance driven by strangers who weren't friendly or helpful. I thought sadly of the two of them waiting together in the emergency room.

I imagined Mr. Sullivan's partner, coming into the hospital to find his companion of so many years cold and forever silent.

I walked for about twenty minutes from the hospital to Central Park. People passed me, talking and laughing, listening to earphones or carrying shopping bags or groceries. Some pushed strollers or walked dogs. There were tourists with cameras, joggers, families walking together. The sun cast long shadows and the fall trees glowed in the late-afternoon light. Beneath the canopy of trees on the border of the park someone called my name and I turned to see Felicity coming toward me with her husband and her mother. At first I couldn't figure out who she was. She looked so familiar and yet I could not place her. I greeted her with a smile and hello and wracked my brain trying to shake off the haze of all the sick patients who were swimming around in my thoughts. Of course. Of course it was Felicity. I had never seen her out of the hospital and there she was, living her life, walking in the park on a beautiful day. It was out of context for me, and it made me laugh to see her; happy to meet her husband who seemed so gentle and handsome and to see her mother, how much Felicity looked like her.

The long hard day faded a little as we stood there chatting, praising the fine weather, talking about what we were doing later that evening. Felicity looked at me closely and asked how the weekend on call had been. I told her that Timothy and his mother had come from Pennsylvania by ambulance and she gave a big sigh. She knew them well.

"Do you think this is the end?" she asked me.

"It's so hard to tell. You know, he's young and there is such resilience."

"But he's bad."

"He's bad, he's really been through so much and they don't want him to get intubated again."

"Oh dear."

"I know. It was hard not to cry. His mother's so nice."

"Oh, I know. Well, here you are."

"Yes. It's a bit disorienting to come from the hospital on a day as beautiful as this. It's almost overwhelming, the contrast with what's going on there." I didn't tell them about sitting with Mr. Sullivan.

"I know. I know what you mean," she said, with her characteristic firm nod of her head up and down.

We parted and they walked south toward the zoo.

My beeper went off. It was the emergency room. I found a quarter in my pocket and went to the corner pay phone. I called the number and was put through to Adam, the medicine resident from our service. He told me that John of the immaculate manicure had another collapsed lung, was oxygenating poorly, and needed admission to the intensive care unit. This time John had been out of the hospital for about four months.

"Adam, listen, on one of his previous admissions the CT surgeons put in a chest tube without giving him anything for pain. They gave him something but didn't wait until it took effect and so he basically had the procedure without pain meds."

"Ouch."

"I'm sure he's afraid that that will happen again."

"Well, he definitely needs another chest tube, but to give him narcotics for it might slow down his breathing too much. Is he DNR?"

"No, he's bounced back pretty well from these episodes so hopefully he will again. He hasn't wanted to make himself DNR. At least not yet. We talked about it recently when he was in clinic. He wants to be on a ventilator if it's necessary."

"Well, we'll make sure to give him something for pain before the chest tube goes in. Hopefully it will go smoothly and he can stay off the vent."

"That would be great. I'll keep my fingers crossed. You'll start him on pentamidine?"

"We already did. Steroids, too."

"Great. I wish he could kick this. It's his third or fourth time getting PCP in the last two years."

"I saw his T cells were twenty-two."

"I know, it's really been a drag. Each time he is a little sicker and it takes him longer to improve."

"Do you want me to call you later?"

"That would be great. Just let me know when he's settled."

I hung up with Adam and wondered if John would survive this hospitalization. Not for the first time I thought about how many times I had seen our patients recover from what seemed like near-death illnesses. So many of our patients were young, and you could not put a value on the capacity of the young body to endure and overcome. But as I walked I also thought of the times when a seemingly stable AIDS patient had taken a sudden turn for the worse and become critically ill within a few hours. AIDS could be so unpredictable. I wondered what course John's illness would take this time around.

Chapter Seven

# 1994 Christmas

"HO-HO-HO that's what I say." He licked his finger and reached around to touch his finger to his behind. "SSSSSSSSSSSSS, oh, I am so hot!" Then he giggled and stood up straight. About six foot six in his size fourteen red spike heels, Darren had on fishnet stockings and a Santa's helper costume. The latter consisted of a white fur-trimmed tutu and a strapless red bodice. He spent a lot of time in the weight room and the muscles in his shoulders bulged. He looked like a bodybuilder trying to disguise himself as a Las Vegas showgirl, complete with a red and white fur-lined Santa cap. "HO-HO-HO, Merry Christmas," he said in a very deep voice.

The secretaries wanted to have their picture taken with him.

Darren wasn't usually a cross-dresser but he loved camping it up at the holidays.

December at the Center for Special Studies meant the patient holiday party. This tradition began when the twenty-fourth floor first opened in 1991. Every patient received an invitation and they came with their families. The big table in the conference room disappeared under all the food. In addition to turkeys, hams, bowls of potatoes and salad, there were enormous piles of sandwiches and cookies, chicken wings, meatballs, and little cocktail hot-dogs. We served soft drinks in the hallway, and the corridor was lined up and down with chairs. The doctors' offices stayed off limits but we left the doors open for the light.

We encouraged the inpatients to come if they could. A nurse or family member escorted them upstairs to the party. Some could walk, some came in wheelchairs. A few of the patients looked like they were ready for the grave. This could be hard on the other guests, knowing that the IV pole, the hospital gown, the gaunt pallor could one day be their own. I remember one Christmas a particularly thin and haggard-looking man sat in a wheelchair in the waiting room, a piece of chocolate cake sagging on a paper plate in his lap. He couldn't eat it. He had a fierce, almost triumphant gleam in his eyes; totally happy to be at the Christmas party. By the look of things it would be his last.

We had a raffle in the first few years of the Christmas party. The hospital, neighborhood stores, and outside charities donated many, many gifts, and Stan or Gerald drew ticket numbers from a box and gave out everything from pen-and-pencil sets to stuffed animals and cologne. Practically everyone got a gift. After a time it became clear that the patients expected a gift and they expected a good one. Sometimes the patients wanted to give their gift back and get something better. Once there was nearly a fistfight over who would get the magenta mule slippers with feathers on them. Grown men fighting over pink mule slippers. We stopped the raffle after that year. But we did continue to give patients gifts for their children.

On the day of the party in 1994 I saw Sophia on my morning rounds. She wore a negligee of see-through pink chiffon and very thick black eye makeup. Twenty-eight years old, Sophia was born Steven, a biological male, but Sophia had lived as a female since the age of fifteen. She took female hormones. She had full, round silicone implants for breasts and silicone injections in her lips as well. She wore glossy pink lipstick and her dark eyes flashed when she smiled. Even in the hospital, even as sick as she was, she projected a sultry sexuality.

"Hello, Dr. Ball," she said in her Lauren Bacall voice.

"Hello, Sophia, how are you feeling today?"

"Better."

"Are you? I'm glad."

"I didn't have no fever."

"Hmmmm." I knew that she'd had a high fever last night but I didn't want to mention it yet. I sat down in the chair next to her bed on top of three folded blue blankets.

"Any news?" she asked.

"No, we're still waiting for the biopsy results."

"I'm scared."

"I know."

"Why does it take so long?"

"Well, it's been just about a week, which is what they usually say. They don't work on the weekends. It's frustrating to wait so long. I know it's hard on you. I called them again last night and I'm hopeful that we'll know something later today."

"OK."

"You didn't eat yet today, did you?" An unopened container of orange juice sat on her tray table. Her breakfast tray had been taken away already.

"I had some breakfast."

"Are you hungry? Today?"

"No. Not really."

She had been losing weight steadily.

"Coughing?"

"No."

"Let me listen to you, OK? Will you sit up for me, please?"

Sophia sat up and leaned forward as I stood and took out my stethoscope. I listened to her back; her lungs were clear. I moved the stethoscope to the front of her chest and listened to her heart. She had a rose tattooed above her left breast. Her heartbeat was fast but steady. I looked in her mouth and felt the lymph nodes in her neck and armpits.

"Well, you certainly sound fine. You did have some fever, though, last night."

"Oh."

"You really don't feel the fevers, do you?"

"Well, sometimes I get completely drenched so then I know."

"But not always."

"No, not always. Do you think it's lymphoma?"

"I know I mentioned lymphoma. But there are other things that cause fevers and weight loss. This could still all be from the MAC," *Mycobacterium avium* complex, an organism that can be found everywhere and is related to tuberculosis but is problematic only in patients who are severely immunosuppressed. "I'm hoping that the lymph node biopsy will tell us later today."

"You can't just treat it without the biopsy?"

"I wish. I wish we could, but the treatments are very different if it's a kind of infection or if it's lymphoma. It's really important to know and I appreciate your patience. I know you'd like to get out of here. I just don't want to say I think you'll go home tomorrow or in three days and then have to turn around and tell you something different. I know the waiting is hard on you but I'm reluctant to send you home with these high fevers and still not have a diagnosis. Hang in there, OK?"

"OK, I will."

"That's great. I'll see you later. Oh, I almost forgot, today is the Christmas party."

"I know, Ronaldo told me."

"Is he coming?"

"I don't know for sure but he's the one who told me about it."

"Well, Sophia, you should come. If you feel like it later, do you want someone to bring you to the party? There's a ton of food and maybe you'd want to eat something at that point."

Her dark eyes sparkled. "I don't really have no clothes."

At this I laughed a little. "Well, see how you feel. Someone could bring you in a wheelchair. Some of the other inpatients are going. One of the clinic patients already showed up in a tutu."

"A tutu?"

"Yes, he's six foot two and wearing high heels."

"Wow." You could see Sophia trying to imagine a six-foot-two male in high heels and a tutu.

"So maybe we'll see you later?"

"What about my hair?" Sophia reached up and held a lock of straight black hair that was resting on her shoulder.

"Your hair?"

"My hair is just awful."

"I think it looks fine." Her hair needed washing but I think mine did too, so I didn't say anything. "I don't think you should not go to the party because of your hair. I hope you'll come."

"Are you going to be there?"

"Of course! The doctors serve the food at this thing. So hopefully I'll see you later." I crossed my fingers as I left, hoping that the biopsy results would not be delayed any longer. Sophia either had something bad or something worse. Most distressing of all would be a negative biopsy result. When there's really something wrong, a negative biopsy result means only that you didn't get the piece of tissue that you needed in order to make the diagnosis. For Sophia that would mean another biopsy, and I fervently hoped that I would not be in a position to have to suggest such a thing to her.

Sophia had been on medication for MAC, *Mycobacterium avium* complex, since her blood cultures revealed the infection three weeks ago. It typically shows up in HIV patients who have fewer than one hundred T cells. The most common symptoms are fevers and weight loss but other symptoms can occur. Some patients become anemic as the MAC organisms invade the bone marrow. Sophia continued to have daily high fevers, often without being aware of them, but by now the fevers due to MAC should have resolved. Something else was going on that gave her the high fevers, poor appetite, and lots of swollen lymph nodes. I worried that she had lymphoma and had mentioned it to her, but until we had the lymph node results I didn't want to have a lengthy conversation with her about this possibility. It wouldn't be fair to talk to her about what it *might* be.

Stan came into the nurses' station while I was writing my note in Sophia's chart. He looked tired. Three patients of his had died in the last week. He'd been very fond of one of them, a guy who used to talk about fishing all the time. I asked him how things were going.

"Fucking Dierdre G. She calls me this morning saying she is going to kill herself. It's about the tenth time she's done this. Why doesn't she do it already and quit fucking bothering me?" Then he gave an exasperated chuckle and groaned. "I called Zoe and asked her if she could squeeze her in this morning."

I had to laugh. Stan could sound so completely irreverent but he was unfailingly compassionate and attentive to his patients. Dierdre G. took up a lot of Stan's time because she was so worried that she was dying of AIDS. Her T cell count remained very high, entirely within the normal range. Unlike my anxious patient Stewart's condition, Dierdre's HIV had not progressed and she really had no medical problems other than neurosis.

"I wish I could give her what she really needs," he said. "I can't write a prescription for a different childhood or a negative HIV test." He looked glum.

"Why is she calling this time?"

"Oh, I don't know, her boyfriend was out too late or her mother said something she didn't like. She knows we can't blow her off if she mentions suicide."

"You're too good to her," I said, shaking my head. "You always listen to her, every time."

"I know, I know." He pulled a maroon chart out of the rack and opened it on the desk along the wall. I recognized the name on the chart as the boyfriend of John of the immaculate manicure.

"So how is Roger?" I asked.

"Oh, he's probably going home tomorrow. Thank God."

"Wow, he was really sick. Good job."

"Yeah, well, the house staff helped a lot on the case. They were great."

A little later at my desk in the clinic upstairs I got a call from the pathology lab. Dr. Annabel Crenshaw, one of the head pathologists, took a special interest in HIV and its many manifestations. Her knowledge and experience were a valuable resource when it came to discussing abnormalities in cells or biopsy results on our patients. Over the phone she told me that Sophia's biopsy results revealed tuberculosis of the lymph nodes.

"She has MAC already, you know," I told her. "Her blood cultures were positive a few weeks ago."

"I know. The sheet had said that. The biopsy showed a lot of organisms so we had to wait for the fixed slides to see the structure. It's pretty classic caseating granulomas. He has both."

"She."

"She. Oh, sorry. It says male on the requisition."

"I know. Her name is Sophia now."

"Well, she has TB."

"OK, well, thanks, Annabel. I was worried that it was lymphoma. This is good news if such a thing is possible. I appreciate your calling."

"You're welcome. Good luck with her."

"Yeah, thanks again." Fortunately, Sophia's chest films showed no disease and she didn't have a cough. This meant that she did not need to be in a respiratory isolation room. The tuberculosis organisms were growing in tissues outside her lungs.

As I put the phone down I thought of my father. On the one hand, my parents were very proud of me. Although I have an older cousin who is a veterinarian, I am the first medical doctor in my family. At first my parents worried about my working with patients with AIDS. They felt alarmed that I might "catch" a "case of AIDS" by working at CSS. I assured them that I didn't intend to share injection drug needles with patients and I wasn't going to have sexual encounters with them either. Once they got over the shock of hearing me say that, they enjoyed learning about the work. They knew about AIDS from the newspapers and television and they took pride in my working in a field of such urgent need. I wasn't in Africa; that also pleased them.

On the other hand, when my father realized that some of the patients we cared for had tuberculosis, he wanted to make sure that my work environment was as safe as it could be. My father sold air filtration systems and worked with large businesses and laboratories to create clean rooms using various combinations of filters and ventilation. Knowledgeable and open-minded, he loved to talk about his work, and his customers liked him because he also knew how to listen. He could talk the blueberries off a muffin but in turn he appreciated a good story and he loved people: hearing about their lives and their families and travels and golf games. He had strongly negative opinions regarding the type of ventilation and filtration at the medical center in the rooms for patients who needed respiratory isolation.

In order for a coughing patient who was suspected of having tuberculosis to be in the hospital, we needed rooms where the airflow didn't spill the airborne germs out into the hallways and the lungs of the other patients and staff. Rooms with reverse or negative ventilation were created so that the airflow would stay within the room and be ventilated out through ducts and filters, not the open door. The rooms we had functioned as they should, but my father worried that they were far from state-of-the-art. He felt that our big, prestigious New York City medical center ought to have better respiratory isolation rooms. He knew of several ways in which the airflow in a room could be directed so that the caregivers would be protected much more thoroughly. The size of the biological matter, whether bacterium, virus, or particle of dust, influenced the type of filter that needed to be in place. The filters in our hospital could not protect us against certain organisms, and my father worried about this.

The medical center had undertaken the construction of an enormous new hospital that would replace most of our current inpatient facilities. My father spoke several times with the engineers regarding the plans for the air filtration and ventilation system. The engineers were agreeable to making changes but ultimately needed direction from the architects and decision makers within the hospital administration. My father was frustrated when the chief epidemiologist of the hospital refused to meet with him to discuss the need for better ventilation systems.

"Well, Suze, you will have a new hospital with a fifty-year-old ventilation design." I thought of these words as I hung up after Annabel's call. Sophia had both MAC and tuberculosis. Because Sophia's TB infection didn't involve her lungs, she wouldn't need respiratory isolation, but my father would still be shaking his head.

As a medical student I learned about tuberculosis as an illness of the third world. As one of the leading causes of death from infectious disease worldwide, it is a fascinating illness with a history dating back thousands of years. Though it is best known as a lung infection, I also learned about the many extra-pulmonary forms of tuberculosis, such as Pott's disease, in which the vertebral bodies are infected: the patient has back pain and may lose the ability to walk. Or pericardial tuberculosis, which can present as if the patient had heart failure. Tuberculosis can also be an infection of the central nervous system or the kidneys or the lymph nodes. In the United States, cases of TB had declined steadily since the early 1900s and it was assumed that most of us would never see a case of it unless we traveled to underserved countries. All these extra-pulmonary forms and more were documented in our texts but were taught more as interesting history than as likely differential diagnoses. Then in the early 1990s, tuberculosis reemerged in New York City as a public health threat.

Two situations contributed to the rise in new cases of tuberculosis in urban centers in the United States in the latter part of the twentieth century. First, the budget cuts of the late 1980s eliminated funding for DOT (directly observed therapy) programs. To treat and cure tuberculosis effectively, patients need to take medication regularly for several months. DOT programs provided a nurse or health worker to actually watch a patient take every dose of his or her prescribed medication. This ensured that patients completed therapy for tuberculosis. Cutting the programs resulted in an upswing of recurrent cases and an increase in cases of drug-resistant tuberculosis in patients whose disease had been incompletely or inadequately treated because they hadn't taken their medications correctly or had discontinued them too soon.

Second, the AIDS epidemic provided a new and vulnerable source of patients, particularly in New York City. HIV infection, regardless of CD4 cell count, placed patients at increased risk to develop TB if they were exposed to it. In patients without HIV infection, fewer than 5 percent of those who are exposed to tuberculosis will actually develop TB in their lifetime. HIV patients, however, have approximately a 5 percent risk *per year* of developing tuberculosis if exposed.

Tuberculosis is well known to occur in groups and clusters where people live close together under inadequately ventilated living conditions. Before I came to CSS, I worked at a different big medical center in another part of New York City, and across the street the city ran a huge men's shelter. At night hundreds of homeless men slept there in cots laid out in rows. We used to think of it as a big petri dish for nascent tuberculosis germs. Because the stain for these organisms turned them red on the slide, we referred to them as red snappers. I had a surreal image of them hopping happily around among the snoring, coughing men in the shelter at night.

Patients with HIV who developed tuberculosis were more likely to have atypical or extra-pulmonary TB. We saw pericardial tuberculosis and tuberculosis of the lymph nodes, TB of the kidneys or tubercular brain abscesses.

What we'd learned as a quasi–history lesson in our textbooks now turned out to be pertinent data for our patient care. With her positive lymph node biopsy, Sophia was my latest patient to be diagnosed with extra-pulmonary tuberculosis. I felt relief at the diagnosis despite a long course of difficult treatment ahead. Even with a concomitant diagnosis of AIDS, tuberculosis could be successfully treated and even cured. Had her biopsy revealed lymphoma, Sophia's prognosis would be much more guarded.

By four thirty that afternoon I was standing behind a long row of steam tables dishing out fried dumplings and rice in one of the big meeting rooms of the hospital cafeteria. My colleagues served up chicken wings and broccoli, macaroni and cheese and salad and little hot dogs and baked fish and beans. On another table heaps of sandwiches sat next to trays of cookies. Patients and their partners, children, and friends, all with plates piled with food, milled about or sat at the many tables each decorated with a red cloth and ribbons and a centerpiece. Christmas music and sometimes dance music played loudly. I looked over to see my enormously obese patient get up out of her wheelchair and start dancing. She had fantastic rhythm and her body gracefully swayed and twisted to the music.

"Celia's out of her wheelchair." Dr. Berry yelled over to me above the noise.

"Lookin' *fine!*" I heard one of the social workers say.

"It's a miracle," I said to Maggie, standing next to me.

Celia wasn't crippled. She was just too fat to move about very easily, so the wheelchair got her where she needed to go, with the help of the home attendant who pushed her everywhere. Someone commented that the home attendant would need a wheelchair herself after pushing Celia around for a few months. Still, I smiled to see my patient on her feet, moving so beautifully.

After the first two or three years, the Christmas party had gotten too big and too crowded for us to continue to have it in the clinic. With patients everywhere, food and drinks invariably spilled on the carpets and the couches. Some patients couldn't see us without asking for a quick visit or a prescription. It was considered bad form to go into your office and shut the door to take a break from the noise or the crowd, but after a couple of hours we all started feeling like we desperately needed the party to be over. We loved hosting the event but it needed a different venue.

The hospital cafeteria did not seem like a warm and welcoming spot for our Christmas party, but we realized the improvement. Much more space for everyone, much more elbow room for eating, talking, and dancing. One of our social workers, Anna, proved to be an excellent DJ, and patients and staff alike were grooving it up on the dance floor. Eventually a karaoke machine became part of the Christmas party. Some of our patients have revealed wonderful voices over the years.

Santa always came to the party, and the kids took turns sitting on his lap telling him what they wanted for Christmas. Darren in his Santa's helper outfit liked to sit on Santa's lap too. Our Santa worked at the local deli and sometimes smelled like he'd been dipping into the eggnog before coming to the party but he proved himself a good sport. He didn't look entirely comfortable with Darren sitting on his lap but he never said whether it was because Darren was wearing a tutu or because Darren weighed 210 pounds.

Suddenly the tempo of the music shifted and there was a general cheer from the dancers. Several people jumped up from their seats to join in the Macarena, a line dance with syncopated moves performed in unison. I watched smiling as the patients and staff as well as kids and assorted friends performed this precise dance all together, struck by the range of enthusiasm. My patient Orlando danced with his head down, wearing cowboy boots, his hair combed back from his face and his shirt nicely pressed. He seemed utterly engrossed in his steps. Several of the secretaries danced together and whooped each time the routine called for the little jump with a turn. Some of the patients danced with exaggerated gestures and great swinging of the hips and arms. Others seemed restrained, almost solemn, going through the movements deliberately, as if participating in a religious ritual.

Out of the blue I thought of Yolanda, my patient with the horrible case of genital herpes. She'd been hospitalized several times this year and died not long ago from overwhelming, untreatable infection. Early in her last, long hospital stay, before she'd become comatose, she'd been able to sit up in a chair for brief periods. The nurses had brought her to the solarium one afternoon, where I went to find her on my rounds. Another patient, a woman in her forties, sat in the bright room with her three visiting children. Yolanda looked on as the kids hummed the music to the Macarena and showed their mother how well they could do the dance. Seeing me, Yolanda asked me to take her back to her room and then didn't speak as I pushed her wheelchair down the hall. Yolanda never talked very much and her silence didn't bother me. When we got back to her room, though, she said, "I liked seeing those little kids do that dance. They seem so free. But then I remembered that I can't do that dance now. I can't even stand up."

She wouldn't say any more to me about it. The nurses told me that she wouldn't go back to the solarium after that. Here I was watching the Macarena again.

One of the people joining the dance was Dierdre G., Stan's patient who had called earlier to say that she was going to kill herself. Zoe Prin stood near me and I asked her if she had met with Dierdre earlier.

"Yeah." She almost hollered above the music and the general din. "Stan asked me to see her and she came in after lunch."

"It looks like you cured her!"

"Oh, you know Dierdre, everything is such a huge trauma. She was at some mall in Staten Island yesterday and she felt like some lady was looking at her in a funny way. She was convinced this woman knew that she has HIV. It totally freaked her out."

"Oh poor Dierdre, she is so tough. Of all people."

"I know, she is totally fine."

"Totally. Stan said she has something like six hundred T cells. So what did you say to her?"

"Well, Stan saw her for a few minutes before I did and I think that settled her down. I just wanted to make sure that her suicidal talk didn't need more intervention. It never does with her but I always like just to check."

"So she's not killing herself today?"

"I invited her to the Christmas party instead. At first she didn't want to come."

"It's good you convinced her. Look at her grooving it up."

Stan walked by us just then. We commented that Dierdre looked pretty great out there on the dance floor. Stan held out both hands as if he were weighing an object in each one. "Hmmmm," he said, "kill myself or do the Macarena? What a hard decision!"

The three of us laughed at how ridiculous that sounded. But we laughed in relief, too, that Dierdre could be out there dancing and we could joke about her dramatics. A patient as medically well as Dierdre frustrated us when so many others needed our care. She might get sick at some point but no one could say when it would happen. One aspect of suffering for Dierdre meant living with that uncertainty. Other patients out on the dance floor moved about like living ghosts, swaying to the music on emaciated limbs, faces lined with the creases of the very ill. I could pick out two or three who would not attend next year's party: Stan's patient sitting in his wheelchair pale as a glass of milk, bony hands and blue veins; my patient Marta, nodding her head to the music, with two of her children sitting close by; her sunken eyes had purple circles around them. Of course, who could know if any one person would survive or not? But AIDS never seemed to let up; despite the youth of the patients and despite the offerings of CSS and our big hospital, too many of those people on the dance floor would not see another Christmas. I shook my head against the feeling of helplessness that crept too close. We needed medicine but sometimes dancing was all we could offer.

# Chapter Eight

# 1995 Another Support Group

The view from my office window on the twenty-fourth floor showed only varying hues of gray on another dreary Thursday morning. As it continued to rain, the sky and buildings blended in the misty air. Warm January temperatures seemed suspicious. I would have preferred that it snow.

"You don't think it's PCP?" Stewart's question drew me back. I had glanced out at the weather while getting a copy of his lab work from the printer by the window.

"I don't think it's PCP." I turned to him as I spoke. I'd already answered this question a few times. Here for a regular clinic appointment, Stewart worried and complained of a dry cough.

"Well, I mean, I don't want to have PCP again." His eyebrows rose up and wrinkled his forehead.

"I'm sure. How long have you had this cough?"

"Well, I think I started to notice it last weekend when we went to Karen's sister's house to watch the football game. I think they have three cats." Stewart wore a clean, pressed shirt and a look of great anxiety. His short, sparse hair, more like gray tufts, needed a comb.

"You were coughing then?"

"I think that's when it started."

"Was it because of the cats? Are you allergic?"

"No, no, I like cats. We have a cat."

"Oh yes, I remember, sorry. I remember that you like cats. So the cough is not from the cats."

"No, I guess not. You remember it was very windy that day? But warm. We were out in Gina's backyard. They had a barbecue and I think it might have been the smoke."

"The smoke made you start coughing?"

"I started coughing then, yes, I think so."

"And are you coughing anything up?"

"No, it's just a dry cough. That's why I'm worried." He cleared his throat. "See? I can't seem to stop it."

"Have you had any fevers?"

"No."

"Do you feel short of breath?"

"When I start coughing I can get short of breath." He held a large pair of aviator sunglasses in his hands and he tapped them on his knee while he spoke.

"Was anyone else coughing from the smoke at the barbecue?"

"Oh, everyone was. My brother-in-law doesn't know how to barbecue and it was so smoky we were all coughing. My clothes smelled like lighter fluid for days." As he said this his face suddenly relaxed and he gave a chuckle. I looked at him and didn't know if I wanted to scream or laugh. I decided on the latter.

"OK, so the smoke from the barbecue made you all cough. Is anyone else still coughing that you know of? Is Karen?"

"I don't think so. You'd have to ask her."

"Are you coughing in the night?"

"No, the cough is only in the day. But, Dr. Ball, I'm really worried. You don't think it's PCP?" His eyebrows remained high up on his forehead.

"Let me listen to you in just a second; it doesn't sound like you have PCP, though, by what you're telling me."

"My T cells are still so low. I, I'm just worried. Dr. Ball, I think I need to be on more medicine."

"You mean more HIV medicine?"

"Yeah. I was reading about a drug that came out that they use with AZT."

"You mean DDI?"

"I forget what it was called, dye-dan something."

"That's probably it. It's a drug named didanosine; we call it DDI. It's being used in combination with AZT and the results are better than just treating with AZT alone."

"DDI. That's the one I heard of. Do you think I could be on that drug? I don't want to get sick again."

I looked at Stewart and considered. Because of his almost hysterical fear of medications, I hadn't ever brought up starting a new drug. Prior attempts had led me into sessions that entailed thirty minutes or more of repetitive questions only to end with him refusing my suggestions. It was now over two years since he'd left the hospital in the middle of his PCP treatment to go to a bar mitzvah in Florida. Despite my advice not to go, he made it there and back without a problem, reporting that he'd even danced the hora alongside his eighty-year-old Aunt Mildred. Once he returned to New York, I struggled to get him to accept a monthly inhaled treatment meant to avoid another bout of PCP. After what felt like much beating of my head against a wall he agreed. He tolerated it without a problem. Now he was asking me to give him a drug that, despite its recent approval for use, we didn't know a lot about. I took it as a significant first step that he was the one to ask for it, but I didn't kid myself that it would be easy. "We could give it a try," I said, with a nod of my head.

"You mean you'd have me start it?"

"It could help get your T cells up. They still are pretty low. The patients who were on DDI with AZT had better increases in their T cells."

"Does it have sulfa in it?"

"No, not that I'm aware of. But I'll double-check to be sure."

"I don't want to have a reaction to it. What are the side effects?"

Inwardly I sighed: here we go; brace yourself. "Some patients up here were in the study. It was well tolerated."

"And they're fine?"

"One patient got some tingling in his toes after being on the drug for several weeks. I think that was the only thing that I've heard of so far. It went away when he stopped taking the DDI."

"Tingling in the toes," Stewart said, almost to himself. "And that was it?"

"I'll double-check with the people down the hall but I think it went pretty well."

"But it might have other side effects." He looked at me with an almost desperate expression on his face.

"It's a new drug, Stewart. Often there are side effects that show up after the drug is approved that we might not have seen at first."

"Do you think it's safe for me?"

"I think if you're interested in being on it, we should give it a try."

"But it might have other side effects, right?"

I wanted to be honest with him but I had that sinking feeling. "That is always a possibility. These drugs don't get approved if they aren't deemed safe, but as you know too well, some people have bad reactions that we don't anticipate."

"Maybe it isn't a good idea."

I resisted the urge to roll my eyes. Instead I watched an imaginary me lean over my desk and grab him by the collar with my two hands and shake him so that his teeth rattled while I shouted a spluttering tirade of frustration into his face. I did allow myself a little shrug. He'd been through such an ordeal with the horrible drug reaction a few years ago. Stewart didn't need reminding that nearly all the skin on his body had painfully burned and peeled off as a result of taking a prescribed drug. Medicine had let him down; I couldn't blame him for being wary of something new.

"Stewart, it's certainly possible that there are side effects that we don't know about. I just can't guarantee that there aren't. The drug did get approved, which means that they studied it in patients and have decided that it's safe and that it can help."

"Would I still take AZT?"

"Yes, you'd stay on your AZT."

"I would take the DDI at the same time? What if they have a reaction together?"

"They were studied together. They are supposed to work together."

"How does it work?"

"Its mechanism is the same as AZT. It inhibits an enzyme of HIV to prevent it from replicating."

"And people had their T cells go up?"

"Patients who took both drugs together did better than patients who took only one drug at a time."

"Can you write me a prescription?"

"I want to clarify for sure that there is no sulfa in it. You're coming back later in the week for your pentamidine, right?"

"I'll be here on Friday."

"We'll talk on Friday. I'm pretty sure it's fine but I want to talk to the study people down the hall and make sure."

"Oh, now I'm worried that I am going to get side effects."

"Listen. I think DDI is a good idea for you and maybe it will help bring up your T cells. If there are any problems with it that I find out about I'll tell you and we won't start it. OK? Now come and sit on the examining table so that I can listen to your lungs." I realized that Stewart had not coughed once during this conversation and he definitely did not seem short of breath. His lungs were clear and the rest of his exam didn't reveal any problems. He asked me a few more times if I thought he had PCP but I stayed firm. After our visit he headed down the hall to see Dr. Prin. I wondered if she had any extra Valium.

Stewart surprised me sometimes with his knowledgeable questions. The information on DDI, for example, had only recently been reported in the lay press and the popular health magazines. Stewart read what he could about HIV and often brought his questions to me. Occasionally his information came from television or radio. Later on it would come from Internet sites, some reliable, some less so. A ranting individual at a Narcotics Anonymous meeting or someone at the organization where he ate lunch might mention a new treatment or test. If Stewart misinterpreted what he read or heard, it could be onerous to try to correct him. I thought of Stan. He had a patient who took things a few steps further, routinely faxing Stan articles on extremely technical or esoteric topics. He'd call ahead to make sure the fax came through so that Stan would be ready for a discussion. Endlessly patient, Stan usually did read or glance through the material, but he admitted that the guy and his reading material could be annoying. "I wouldn't mind it so much if the articles were interesting," he said one day. "But they are the most boring, ridiculously tedious pieces of information. Why can't he send me something relevant? Or even irrelevant, I don't care, just a little bit interesting." Stan and I could always successfully waste a few minutes in the hall complaining to each other.

I knew that when Stewart returned on Friday I'd probably have the same conversation as today regarding DDI. He'd ask about the possible side effects and the risk of allergic reaction. He'd probably have a lot more to say about toe tingling at that point. I made a note to reread the available information on DDI and review the potential side effects.

Stewart took AZT but he knew, as did we all, that it probably wasn't helping him. After six years on the market, it seemed clear that patients on AZT didn't have a better survival rate than those off it. The data from the Concorde study, presented in Berlin in 1993, had demonstrated AZT's lack of impact on mortality. Patients taking the drug did not report improved symptoms, but more important, the transient rise in T cells from taking AZT didn't translate into patients' living any longer. Arguments went back and forth about details of the study but the bottom line was that we hadn't made any progress in treating patients with AIDS. The study merely confirmed our clinical experiences.

I thought of Peaches, who made me chuckle with her raucous laughter and her itchy belly, sitting in my office saying, "I ain't takin' that shit." I hadn't seen Peaches in a while. She never took the AZT that I'd prescribed. I could fault her data source but in the end I could not fault her decision.

As I was speaking to Stewart that morning, Stan received a call that his mother, in Virginia, had metastatic ovarian cancer. When I walked past his office on the way to the lab, he waved me in as he was getting off the phone with one of his patients. He'd already called the airlines and had a reservation on a flight later in the evening. I sat down and went through his inpatient list with him, not an easy task for Stan, who couldn't concentrate and looked flustered and pale. I'd been on call the previous weekend and already knew most of the people he had in the hospital. "Just go," I said, taking the paper from him. He surprised me when he said that he wanted to finish making his calls and go to support group that afternoon.

I went out to the waiting room to call in my next patient. She sat in a comfortable chair by the wall. Her spaghetti-strapped camisole was having a hard time containing her ample bosom. The rose tattoo sat provocatively on her left breast. As she gracefully stood up and walked across the room toward me, I saw that there were several pairs of eyes following her movements. Her dark eyes sparkled and her silicone-enhanced lips glistened bright pink.

"Hello, Dr. Ball," she said in her sultry Brooklyn-accented voice.

"Look at you, Sophia," I said, smiling. "Come on in."

We went into my office and sat down.

"Sophia, you look fantastic."

"Thank you, Dr. Ball."

"How much weight have you gained?"

"I think about fifteen pounds."

I kept staring at her and smiling. "And you feel good?"

"Yes, I'm doing good now."

"How many months of treatment do you have left?"

"I just got my second refill at the pharmacy last week. I think I need five more after that."

"Terrific. You'll stay on the Rifabutin and the Myambutol as well, and stay on your Bactrim, too."

"Yeah, I know, Jean went over it with me." Jean was our homecare nurse. She played the critical role of ensuring that our discharged patients made a safe and stable transition from inpatient to home. As a former visiting nurse, she took into consideration the details of patients' living conditions such as how many stairs to the front door, would there be room for the home attendant, was there access to food. She also made sure the patients understood their medication lists and that the local pharmacies had the necessary prescriptions. Jean's job was part doctor, part social worker, and we all depended on her, patients and providers alike.

"That's great. How are you doing otherwise?"

"I'm doing good. I want to get back to one sixty. I'm eating much better."

"And you restarted the estrogen a few weeks ago, right?"

"Yeah."

Sophia had to swallow or be injected with a whole slew of various compounds to treat her double infections with MAC and tuberculosis. Initially she'd experienced a lot of side effects and complications. The days dragged on. Still, she didn't have lymphoma, which would have involved chemotherapy and a significantly poorer prognosis, and we encouraged Sophia to hang in there. It seemed to take forever but she slowly turned around. Her fevers diminished, she began to eat a bit, she got up and walked around, she did her nails. Now here she sat in my office looking like a candidate for a magazine that your uncle might hide under the bed. Success!

Sophia still had AIDS. It occurred to me that we rarely saw our patients bounce back to health when they had AIDS. I couldn't tell what Sophia's future course would be. For all she'd been through she remained vulnerable to whatever AIDS threw at her. All the same, I appreciated the small victory of this moment.

"Dr. Ball, what happened to Geraldine?" She was asking about a patient of Maggie's whom she'd gotten to know when they'd both been hospitalized at the same time.

"Geraldine died a few months ago."

"Oh."

In the clinic we knew Geraldine as a lovely woman, very fastidious about her makeup and her clothes. She'd been born a he, a boy named Jerry until she changed it more than ten years ago. Sophia and Geraldine met and became friends in the hospital, bonding over their common history. They also had similar pink silk bathrobes and wore fluffy slippers. I remembered seeing them sitting in the solarium together, looking through *Vogue* magazine. Geraldine sported a turban and Sophia had some sort of wispy scarf wrapped around her head. When I asked if they were having bad hair days they laughed.

Geraldine's illness progressed after Sophia went home. Sophia did not see the debilitation of those last several weeks as Geraldine became increasingly weak and eventually could not move from her bed or even feed herself. Her weight plummeted and she spent most days drifting in and out of consciousness. The estrogens in her body diminished without the regular hormone injections and the biological levels of testosterone returned. Her voice deepened. Since she could no longer attend to her daily cosmetic regime, with its close shaving and pancake makeup, a fine, soft beard began to cover her chin and hollow cheeks, and her plucked, arched eyebrows grew back. The features of her nose coarsened and changed. It was as if Jerry had come back to reclaim his face from Geraldine.

Maggie spoke one day in support group of watching this slow metamorphosis of one person into another. I remember seeing Janice shake her head sadly as we all listened to this macabre tale. Geraldine had created something fine and precious for herself. AIDS had come along and slowly destroyed her creation. As if the ocean, with all its tides and seasons, was reclaiming its coastline after someone had built a lovely glass palace on the water's edge.

Sophia did not ask me any more questions about what happened to her friend. I wondered if she might have some idea or have heard from others what Geraldine had looked like in the end. Sophia had had a reprieve. She had recovered. Her friend did not. We didn't talk about it any further.

After Sophia left and I put down some notes in her chart, I went out to the waiting room and called Bella in. My happiness with Sophia's recovery faded quickly as I spotted Bella's disheveled form across the waiting room. Things were going badly with Bella: she was getting sicker by the day. I couldn't know then that I'd be dealing with Stewart's anxiety and Sophia's sultry flirtations for years to come but there was little time left with Bella, a woman for whom I felt much respect though I'd known her only briefly.

Bella and her husband, Cecil, had contracted HIV by sharing heroin needles. Both had very advanced disease. They adored their two sons, Nathan and Jason, but in their worry and their guilt they had told neither boy about their infections. Nor had they told the younger son, Jason, that he too carried the virus. The older boy, Nathan, knew only that his brother had a blood disorder requiring a lot of doctors' appointments and medications and that his parents struggled with drug use. He'd seen them shoot up together in the bathroom of their apartment. When he was ten and Jason was four, Bella finally gave up drugs for good. She stayed clean but her HIV progressed. She had the support of a brother and sister who pitched in to care for the boys when she couldn't. Lately, Bella needed to be hospitalized with increasing frequency. Several episodes of bacterial pneumonia resulted in her losing weight and depending more and more on her siblings for help. Still, she didn't tell her older son. We talked to both parents about needing to tell Nathan so that the boy could have some time to think about his parents' and brother's illness and prepare for what might be coming. Bella and Cecil really loved each other. Neither blamed the other for what had happened. Both carried profound grief and guilt at having a son with HIV. They knew, too, that soon they would have to tell Nathan. They so wanted to spare him, to protect him. He knew something was wrong, but meanwhile Nathan led a busy fifteen-year-old boy's life.

Cecil, the boys' father, continued to struggle with drug use. He wanted to stop but admitted that the drugs helped him forget briefly that he had AIDS and his wife and son also had AIDS. He suffered from terrible rashes that no one could figure out. He got his HIV care at another clinic but I knew from Bella that his T cell count was very low. One day he came to Bella's visit with her and told me he wished it were all just a bad dream, and that he could wake up and have their happy family once again.

Bella came into my office, sat down, and started to cough. Her dry, straw-colored hair hung about her face and her hands were red, with bitten, stubby nails. She wore a clean work shirt and a pair of corduroy pants. She did not wear makeup, her teeth looked bad, and her eyes had dark circles under them. She put her hand on her chest as she coughed. Clearly it hurt.

"Hi. You don't look like you feel very well."

She shook her head, still coughing with her hand on her chest, her eyes closed.

"Have you had fevers?"

"Yes," she said finally, after coughing up something large and wet into a tissue. "The last two nights it was a hundred and two. And chills. Oh, it hurts so much when I cough." She had tears in her eyes.

"Oh, Bella." I looked at her unhappily, thinking she needed to come into the hospital again. "How are the boys?"

"They're OK. My sister came and got them this morning. They'll go to her house after school. Jason has a doctor's appointment tomorrow morning. He's been doing good, though."

"And Nathan?"

"Nathan's playing football."

"How is that? Does he enjoy it?"

"Oh he loves it. He's a tight end. He has a girlfriend."

"That's great. Is he practicing safer sex?"

"He better be!" She started to cough again. "I told him he has to."

"Did you tell him why?"

"Well, no. But I think he's not doing it. I don't think he's ready. I think sex is still too, too not for him. He's interested but he's pretty shy."

"But he knows about condoms, right?"

"We both talked to him, Cecil and me. We told him that we didn't want no girls getting pregnant. I don't think he's doing it."

"But you didn't tell about you or Cecil or Jason? Or about condoms as a protection from getting or transmitting HIV?"

"No. Not yet." She looked down at her chapped hands and twisted her wedding ring.

"I know that you're working on this. It's hard. How's Cecil?"

"Getting high."

"Oh boy."

"He's really down these days. This rash is killing him. I think he's going to come here instead. He wants to come see you."

"Well, that's fine. I'm sorry he's using though."

"It's so hard for him. He wants to leave it but then he gets so down and he goes out for a walk and then he doesn't come back."

"What do you say to the boys?"

"Jason will still ask where's Daddy but Nathan knows. He don't even ask no more." She started to cough again, holding her chest. I watched from across my desk, knowing that Bella would not survive this, feeling as if she were getting farther away from me even as we sat there. The distance between us made me squint to see more clearly. I realized that I had also put my hand on my chest. I pictured Bella and Cecil in a bathroom, Bella sitting on the toilet and Cecil on the edge of the tub. Bella held the spoon and the tiny syringe while Cecil placed a tourniquet below a rolled-up sleeve. I pictured a little boy in Batman pajamas knocking on the door, sleepily calling for Mama. It took me a moment to shut out the overwhelming sense of sadness as Bella sat in my office and coughed, her dry straw hair covering her face.

"Bella," I said, "you are too sick to go back home today."

She nodded as she coughed and I saw tears on her cheeks.

"Do you want me to call Cecil to let him know? Or your sister?"

"My sister," she said between coughs. "Cecil will call her later if I'm not home."

I walked Bella down the hall to a room where she could lie down. I examined her, noting the fever and the clattering sounds in her lungs, and then

I spoke to the nurses to order her blood tests and chest X-ray. I called the admitting office and the bed resident to tell them about the admission. I thought about what I sensed was in store for Bella and probably for Cecil as well. How hopeful it had seemed to have Sophia stroll into my office after her many weeks in the hospital. Even Stewart, exasperating as he was, had made it home from Florida and his nephew's bar mitzvah and back to CSS. Seeing the patients both in and out of the hospital provided a much fuller understanding of their lives. The residents saw the AIDS patients only in the hospital, which distorted their view. Bella would be pathetic and sick in their eyes. I knew Bella for her loving way with her kids, her subtle, self-deprecating humor, and her funny, cheap hair dye efforts to be a blonde. I hoped she'd make it back to see me as an outpatient. AIDS magnified the continuity of seeing a patient over time. I couldn't know or guess how long I would be caring for patients like Stewart and Sophia, or crack-loving Peaches, or independent Etta, with her little son Joey. AIDS could make people very sick very fast, so our continuity felt all the more hard-won and special.

By the time we sat down around the big table in the conference room later, almost everyone knew that Stan had received very bad news. Dr. Jacobs sat in his usual chair against the wall. He looked at the floor as he normally did but his brow had an extra crease. Stan sat in a chair at the table but he rested his elbows on his knees and he too looked at the floor.

Janice did not wait for a long communal silence to start the session that day. "Stan," she said, "Dr. Jacobs told me before we came in about your mom."

"Yeah," said Stan looking up at her briefly.

"You're going down to see her?"

"Yeah, I'm going down tonight."

"Is there anything we can do?"

He looked up again and covered his mouth with his hand, thinking. "No, I . . . no," he finally said.

Dr. Berry spoke with sadness and concern in her voice. "Will you let us know if we can do anything?"

He looked over at her. "It's just sudden. I have to see. I'll know more tomorrow." He stared at his hands, now clasped on the table.

Clearly Stan and his mother were close. He cleared his throat and said that he was trying not to think the worst despite knowing that her diagnosis meant potential disaster. Sadness often filled that room when the support group met, but today it felt much more personal. I think Dr. Jacobs had met Stan's mother and perhaps Jean and Suzette had as well. Her illness, Stan's sadness touched everyone.

Several people offered him encouragement. He would be a tremendous help to his mother both in getting her the best available medical care and simply by being present for her. Maggie told Stan that she would miss him while he was in Virginia but that she envied Stan's mother. She dabbed at her eyes with a wet tissue. Then, as there was a groan around the table, she realized what she had said. "I mean I don't envy her, but I envy her," she said, flustered. "She'll have you," Maggie said, looking at Stan.

"You have to know that you are the glue around here," said Randall. Randall had been a social worker for many years and worked with Dr. Jacobs long ago in the one-room office that constituted the AIDS clinic at the medical center before CSS. What he said rang true. Purely by example Stan kept us together, as individuals and as a dedicated group. I thought about how much I appreciated his compassion and humor as well as his straightforward clinical approach. He sustained us all with his dedication and his occasional four-letter word. Dr. Jacobs relied heavily on Stan's consistency and clear-eyed perspective; the hospital politics and managerial responsibilities were very much easier for him to bear with Stan's advice and assistance.

Support group shifted a bit that day, taking on a different vantage point as we identified with Stan's sadness and the gravity of his mother's illness. Yet what we talked about, what seemed important to convey, was not how we felt about Stan's mother but how we felt about Stan. Years later this particular session would be remembered by all of us. An unexpected moment in which we recognized how much Stan gave us, how he kept us sane, and we tried to give something back. No doubt anyone in the room with an illness in the family would be well supported by this group. But our response to Stan voiced an acknowledgment of how much he meant to us.

I understood then what Stan already knew—that this group could be our safety net, a place to catch us and help us process some of the acute emotions that we experienced as part of our daily work. He wasn't looking for an outpouring of adoration but he could use the collective emotional support to bolster his courage and his strength. Another person might hesitate to expose such personal and overwhelming feelings, but I saw that Stan drew from our response as if from a well. We often spoke here of our efforts to separate our work from our lives, to avoid carrying outside the misery that crowded our rounds and our office hours. With these colleagues we could be emotionally naked without being embarrassed or afraid. The sustenance in this room did not have to be just for work. Stan knew that.

Janice watched the faces around the table that day as we didn't talk about our patients or HIV or the frustrations of the hospital. Of all the support groups and all the tears and heartache that we brought to that table over the months and years, it seemed ironic yet fitting to be so engaged with Stan and one another over someone who wasn't our patient.

Before leaving for the day, after the support group was over and I'd finished my chart notes and wished Stan a safe trip, I returned a call from a pharmacy that had phoned earlier with a question about Hank. When I got the pharmacist on the line he asked me if I'd ordered a certain medication. He had in his hand a prescription, signed with my name, for a powerful narcotic at a very large dose and quantity. I would never have prescribed it. The pharmacist on the phone chuckled as he said, "Oh that Hank. This is not the first time he's tried to put one over on us. Last week he tried to get some Dilaudid, saying that his prescription had been stolen on the train. I feel bad for the guy but he's not doing himself any favors."

I thanked the pharmacist for calling. Hank hadn't kept an appointment in several months and I wondered if he just accepted that I would not be giving him a prescription for the narcotics he sought. It seemed he'd decided to write his own. The pharmacist clarified that the prescription came from a generic pad, not my personal prescription pad. I asked him to please tell Hank, if he saw him again, to call us for an appointment. I made a note of this call to put in his chart. Forging prescriptions could get a patient kicked out of clinic. Stealing prescription pads could get a person arrested. I guessed we'd discuss it if Hank ever showed up again. Still, I couldn't help but smile at the memory of Hank coming out of the bathroom that day naked but for the toilet paper stuffed in his ears and nose and wrapped around his penis.

# Chapter Nine

# 1995 Mothers and Children

Down the hall from my office a woman stood talking with Jean outside the lab. I didn't recognize her as a patient but she looked familiar to me: a well-dressed woman with brown hair and wire-rimmed glasses; not someone who worked in the hospital, either. As she spoke to Jean and put her hand on her arm, Jean reached out and gave the woman a hug. I walked down the carpeted hallway toward them and, getting closer, I realized that the woman was Timothy's mother, Mrs. Olsen. Perhaps she had come up to visit Jean while Timothy was off at a test. For a moment I felt confused. Timothy had no more tests to go to. He had died months ago and his mother had been with him. I remembered seeing a couple of the nurses crying at the nurses' station that day. Dr. Jacobs had come over from his office to see Mrs. Olsen when it happened. This was my first time seeing her since then. I felt a sudden urge to go back into my office. I didn't know if I could face her sadness. My step slowed a bit but I kept moving forward.

"Dr. Ball, how are you?" She turned toward me and I could tell she was trying to smile.

"Mrs. Olsen." I reached out and hugged her. "It's so nice to see you. I'm so sorry." She hugged me back and over her shoulder Jean was wiping a tear from her cheek. Oh, Mrs. Olsen, what you have seen, what you have been through. I tried to swallow the big lump in my throat.

"I had to come to get some papers and I stopped by to see Dr. Jacobs in his office so I thought why not come up here and see you all as well."

"That is so nice of you," said Jean.

"How are you doing?" I asked her.

"Well, there are definitely good days and bad days. I can't say I miss spending every day in the hospital. But everyone was so nice."

"Oh" was all I could think of to say, looking at her. "We miss him."

"Yes. I miss him too." We stood there looking at one another. Timothy was gone.

"Are you staying in the city?" I asked.

"Tim's brothers are helping me organize his things. His friends, too, have been very helpful."

"You are really kind to come and say hello."

"I wanted to say hello to his nurse Peggy, but when the elevator door opened I just found that I did not want to get off there."

Jean and I both nodded.

"I hope you'll tell her that I stopped by. She was so sweet with Timothy. The others, too, Judy and Angela. They were really great."

"I think Peggy had a crush on Timothy," said Jean, smiling. "I know I did." Her eyes were shining.

Mrs. Olsen laughed a bit. There were sad little lines under her eyes and she'd lost some weight. "Are you taking care of yourself?" I asked her.

"I'm all right," she said. "It was very rough but I am doing all right now. The boys are helping me and he's not suffering anymore."

"No."

I quickly hugged Mrs. Olsen again and walked back down the hall to my office. I thought about that weekend on call when I had seen her with Timothy in the emergency room. What an ordeal they had been through, coming from Pennsylvania by ambulance. So worn out then, very close to the end of the bigger journey. I went into my office and stood looking out the window behind my desk. Without thinking about it my hand went to my belly. I was thinking about mothers and sons. I still couldn't believe it sometimes. My pregnancy felt momentous and wonderful but that thrill immediately gave way to worry. Would my baby be OK? Would it be healthy? Would it survive? I thought of Timothy and that day in the emergency room, how his mother had looked at him. Tears blurred the view out the window. I couldn't imagine what she'd gone through and I ached with the hope that I would never have to. Mothers should not bury their sons. I shook my head and went back to the hall to find the next patient.

The chart in the box outside my door seemed very light, the chart of a woman named Pat, whom I'd seen only once before. I had a mental image of a small, dark-skinned woman who had very pink gums and no teeth. Her drug detox program had set up her appointment and she'd come in to see me the first time with a social worker from the facility. Sullen and hard to interview, she did not want to be living in the detox center and spoke resentfully to the person who'd come with her. Today I read the previous note and realized that four months had passed. She'd missed three follow-up appointments. The labs in her chart showed a T cell count of 122.

I called Pat in and stood in the doorway of the waiting room looking at the patients bustling around. Piles of coats competed with patients for space on the couches; several people leaned over the receptionists' counter waiting to check in or check out; others were gathered at the food shelf, buttering bagels or pouring milk into coffee. A couple of occupied wheelchairs blocked the path to the elevator. After I called Pat's name again a small person who'd been slumped in a chair near the far wall by the elevator raised her head. She got up slowly and came toward me through the crowd wearing a big black coat and a wool hat. She didn't look at me or speak to me as she approached. I held the door open for her and we walked together toward my office.

"Hi, Pat, I'm glad you came back."

"Yeah, well I'm pregnant." We reached the door of my office and I stepped back to let her go in ahead of me. Way down the hall Mary Rose was looking at us, mouthing something to me and pointing to her head and lifting up her hand. Then she pointed to Pat. I followed Pat into my room and sat behind my desk.

"How many weeks pregnant are you?" I asked her.

"I'm about three months." She whistled a little as she spoke and her lips protruded flabbily in front of toothless gums. Her dark coat engulfed her and the maroon knitted hat covered her eyebrows. She looked thin.

"Is this a pregnancy that you want to keep?"

"'Course I want to keep it. I wanna get a 'partment."

"I'm sorry to have forgotten but do you have other kids?"

"My one daughter lives with my mother. She'll be sixteen next month." She pronounced it "monf." I quickly calculated that Pat had been pregnant as a fifteen-year-old and had never returned to school.

"Have you had other pregnancies?"

"I had abortions and miscarriages. One baby died when it was two." Pat pulled out her purse and started rummaging around in it. She relayed the information as if telling me her phone number.

"When did that happen?"

"Oh, I don't know. Maybe five, six years ago."

"Are you involved with the father of this pregnancy?"

She snorted and looked at the ceiling for a moment as if trying not to tell me that she thought my question was one of the more stupid things she'd heard that day. "No," she said. "Here's the papers for you to fill out," and she pulled some crumpled and dirty folded sheets from her purse and handed them across to me.

I took the papers and looked at them briefly. From their wrinkled, torn, and grimy state I could tell that she had been carrying them around for a while. I wondered if she'd even looked at them, as no name or patient information had been written on any of them. One form requested supplemental nutrition allowance and another wanted information to apply for housing. A third form needed medical information for disability.

"Where are you living now?"

"In the shelter. But 'cause I'm pregnant, I get a 'partment."

"Have you seen the obstetricians?"

"Molly's taking me down there later for a 'pointment."

"Are you feeling all right?"

"Yeah, I feel OK." She didn't look at me. I could see cigarettes in her purse.

"So where have you been? Why didn't you come back?"

"I was busy."

"Have you been using?"

"A little. I used a little. If I get my own apartment I won't be using. The shelters is full of drugs."

"Well, we did your labs the last time you were here and your T cells are pretty low."

"How low?"

"A hundred and twenty-two."

She snorted again. "They was ninety before."

"So they're a little better. That's great. Still, they're on the low side and you need to be on some medicine to protect you against PCP. That's a kind of pneumonia."

"I know what PCP is. I was on that medicine before."

"You took Bactrim before?"

"Yeah. My doctors at St. Bernard's gave it to me."

"You haven't had PCP, right? At least that's what you told me last time."

"I had pneumonia."

"Was it PCP?"

"I don't know."

"When was the last time you took Bactrim to protect you from PCP?"

"I don't know. Why are you asking all these questions for? Isn't it in my chart?"

"I don't have any records from St. Bernard's. I just have what you told me from a few months ago when you came here for the first time."

"Damn it's hot in here," she said, shrugging out of her coat and pulling off her knitted hat, revealing an enormous sutured gash that ran across her entire forehead.

"Oh my gosh, Pat, what happened to you?" I sat staring at her forehead; there must have been forty stitches there.

"I got cut." She touched her forehead with her fingers and pushed her hair off her brow.

"You got cut? By a knife?" I knew my question sounded utterly ridiculous; I couldn't help it. I kept staring at the wound. It looked clean, fortunately, not infected or puffy or red. Just huge. This must have been what Mary Rose's gesticulations meant. "When did this happen? Who did this to you?"

"About a week ago. I was in a guy's car and instead of paying me he took out his knife and cut me. Then he was mad because I was bleeding all over his damn car."

"Was it someone you knew?"

"Dr. Ball." She crossed her arms and looked at me with her head cocked to one side. "I was doin' him, OK?"

"Oh."

"Asshole," she said looking away again. "Didn't even pay me. I got him back, though."

"You got him back?"

"I cut his fool face right back. Then I got out of there."

Holy shit, I thought. "Wow," I said.

"Yeah, well, just fill out those papers so's I can get a 'partment. I'm pregnant. I know that qualifies me. Just fill 'em out."

At that point I did not want to argue or discuss her papers with her. She told me that she had an appointment in the surgery center at St. Bernard's in a few days to have her stitches removed. I wanted her to get to today's OB appointment. She needed to start taking AZT, since recent studies had shown that its use in pregnancy could reduce the risk of transmission of HIV from the mother to the fetus, but I'd let the obstetricians write that prescription. In fact, she needed Bactrim, too, with those low T cells, but Bactrim shouldn't be given in the third trimester. The obstetricians should be the ones to write any new prescriptions for her at this point. I made a little note to call them and stuck it on my phone.

Molly came into my office to take Pat down to her OB appointment. She had actually met Pat previously when she was working in the OB clinic and Pat had come in for a pregnancy termination.

"Whoa, Pat! Shit! What happened?" Molly rarely beat around the bush. "Nuthin'."

"OK, well if that's nothin' I'm sure glad something didn't happen. Come on with me and we'll go down to see Dr. La Grangia." Molly looked back at me as they left the room and she mouthed another "holy shit."

I sat at my desk for a moment gathering my thoughts. I felt a little shaky. Without success I tried not to picture what must have happened in that car with an unknown man wielding a knife. Sex for money for drugs. And a pregnancy that didn't mean a baby, it meant an apartment. She spoke of her daughter and the death of a little child with no more emotion than someone talking about a bus schedule; even less. As if they had no importance to her whatsoever. Her pregnancy wasn't about a family; it was about benefits. My hand rested on my belly once again. I had less than three months to go. I'd gone through quite a lot to get pregnant. Having a female partner instead of a husband forced us to be quite deliberate. No happy accident from a romantic evening for our procreative efforts. I'd undergone special tests and studies and lots of drugs. We'd even gotten FedEx involved. It made me incredibly happy when, at twenty weeks, the CSS crew had cheered when I'd told them the news. To general hilarity I told them we'd just stopped using condoms.

Mary Rose came and stood in my doorway.

"So you saw what was under the hat?"

"Oh my gosh. That was unbelievable," I said.

Mary Rose was smiling and shaking her head. "I said to her, 'Pat, what happened?' and she said, 'I got sliced.' So I asked her, 'What did you do?' and she said, 'I sliced him back!'" Mary Rose was laughing and it made me smile too. I realized how unnerved I felt at Pat's misadventure. But Pat wasn't unnerved. She took it in stride. Her life meant facing risks like this every day. Her drug use took her to places that were beyond my reach or understanding and she was trying to make the most of her circumstances. She lived within five miles of where I sat and yet it was as if we were on different planets. Our lives, our language, our food, our culture; we had entirely different ways of life. I thought of Pat as living on the margins of society. But that was *my* perspective. No doubt from Pat's perspective it was me living on the margins. I could condemn her drug use or her utilitarian approach to pregnancy but I had to appreciate and admire her pluck. She wasn't looking for sympathy from me or anyone else. I was just a tool for her, a means to an end; another wagging finger she had to get past to achieve her goals.

"You think he's the father?" Mary Rose asked me.

"Mr. Slice-and-Dice? I doubt it."

"I guess we'll never know, shall we?"

"Damn, what a story."

From the hall we could hear someone singing in a deep, melodious voice. I recognized an excellent imitation of a Lou Rawls song. Mary Rose leaned her head back out the door to see who it was. "You've got to see this," she said to me.

I went to the door to look out and see the singer, but by the time I got there the voice had stopped. I saw only a very tall woman in a tiny, tight miniskirt walking away from us toward the lab. She had remarkably large shoulders and she wore red patent leather shoes that must have had at least six-inch heels. She got to the door of the lab and turned to go in. In a loud, deep voice she said, "Jean, are you ready for me?" and then she laughed a big, booming laugh.

"That would be Darren," I said.

"Lovely voice," said Mary Rose and she went back down the hall herself.

I went out to the waiting room to call my next patient, Olive. I wondered if she would have a new mysterious ailment to tell me about today. It occurred to me as I called her name that Olive never came in the middle of the day; she always arrived first thing in the morning. I looked around the room but didn't see her. One of the people in a wheelchair started moving across the room toward me and I realized with a double-take that it was Olive sitting in the chair. A purple fur jacket lay in her lap as she expertly maneuvered the wheelchair through the chairs in the waiting room. Oh dear, I thought to myself. She had matching purple pumps on her feet, resting on the wheelchair footrests.

We went to my office and I held the door open for her as she wheeled herself into the room. "Olive, what happened? Why are you in a wheelchair?"

"It's my dystonia. I can't walk."

"Did you fall or hurt yourself?"

"No, my muscles don't work. I can't stand up. My legs won't hold me. The doctor told me I should use the wheelchair and not try to get up. I couldn't get up anyway. My legs are too weak."

"Which doctor told you?"

"The doctor on the plane."

I waited for her to go on. I remembered seeing something about dystonia in her chart. She'd never mentioned it and I hadn't asked her about it; there were so many other things on her problem list. Obviously her ears didn't have anything to do with her being in a wheelchair. No; I was thinking of dysphonia. Dystonia meant muscle tone, poor muscle tone.

"I was coming back from Hawaii."

"Oh yes, I remember, you were going to Hawaii with your mother. How was your trip?"

"It was beautiful. I brought in some pictures for you to see. We went to the volcano. But then I got sick." She reached around to a purse that hung off the back of the wheelchair and brought it into her lap.

"You got sick while you were on the trip?"

"The day before we came home I started feeling weak. And then on the plane I couldn't walk. I couldn't get up out of my seat. They had to carry me off when we landed."

"And there was a doctor on the plane who took care of you?" Did I really want to hear this story? Olive was well dressed as always and wore stockings and nice pumps. Her hair had been dyed almost yellow, and elaborately woven tight braids with amber-colored beads wound around her head.

"The doctor came to see me when they announced that one of the passengers needed to see a doctor. He was very nice. From Massachusetts. He examined my legs and told me I should not try to walk."

"And did he say what was wrong with you?"

"Dystonia."

"Your same dystonia from before? Did you tell him that you've been diagnosed with dystonia in the past?"

"Yes. And he said I should get a CAT scan when I get back and see you."

"Have you spoken to Dr. Resh about this? How long have you been back?"

"We got home Tuesday. I called the neurology office and Dr. Resh called me yesterday. I'm going there after this."

"Is your mother still here? I remember you said that you hadn't seen her in a long time."

"She went back to Arizona Wednesday."

"I thought you'd said . . ." I didn't finish. Olive was shaking her head.

"She was going to stay with us for a longer time but when we got back she said she missed her house and wanted to go home to Arizona. So she did."

I nodded, looking at Olive. There was something about her mother. I couldn't remember exactly what it was. "OK, so you can't walk but you don't have pain or numbness. Is that right?"

Olive nodded. She looked relaxed and unfazed by her inability to walk. I got up from behind my desk and went around to where she sat in the wheelchair. I took her blood pressure and looked in her eyes and her mouth. I tested the strength in her hands, arms, and shoulders. I looked at her legs and felt the pulses in her feet. I had her lift one leg and then another, flex the left hip then the right, wiggle her toes, flex and extend her ankles. I tested her reflexes at her elbows and knees. Everything was normal. I ran the base of my reflex hammer along the bottom of her foot looking for a Babinski response. I tested the strength of her lower extremities. She had weakness in her legs, but weakness is notoriously subjective. If you don't make any effort you can appear very weak. How much of Olive's weakness was real? When I lifted up one foot to straighten the leg at the knee, I told her to hold up her foot. At first she held it but then let it drift back down. It didn't flop down. When I asked her to lift her thigh against my hand she seemed to make no effort whatsoever to do so. She had good muscle tone and when I had her close her eyes she withdrew her foot or her leg when I poked her gently with a pin. She easily discerned the difference between the poke of a pin and the touch of my finger. She appeared to have no strength in her legs when asked to exert any effort. The rest of her exam seemed entirely normal. I'd been taking care of Olive for a few years now and I couldn't suppress my skepticism.

But for the inconsistencies in her strength, I found no neurological deficit. Still, I needed the neurologist to take a look and see what he thought. Dr. Resh knew Olive and had treated her in the past for headaches and, now I remembered, for the diagnosis of dystonia. When Olive went to the neurology clinic a few years ago Dr. Resh told her that her symptoms came from illness related to her HIV. I called him and assured him that Olive's immune system functioned well and that her HIV was not the source of her problems, at least not yet. I gave him some of her history, the long workups for problems that eventually disappeared on their own. "Ah," I remember him saying, "there is some somatization here that presents from time to time, if I understand you correctly." I appreciated that he understood Olive and continued to see her himself rather than having a different resident see her every time she went to the clinic. He addressed each problem as it presented; he did not order a vast array of tests. I wondered what his conclusion would be after seeing her this afternoon.

"Did you already see Dr. Prin today?"

"Yes. And I showed her my pictures, too."

"Did she comment at all on your inability to walk?"

"She said to talk to you and to Dr. Resh."

"Great. Well, I don't have a clear answer for you right now. I'm not sure a CT scan would be that helpful but I'll wait to see what Dr. Resh would like to do. I'll give him a call later."

Olive looked into her purse and brought out a glossy folder that had a palm tree on it. Inside there were several photos of Olive in evening wear standing with a shorter older woman. They had their arms around each other and they each had a cocktail in one hand with an umbrella in it. They were smiling at the camera. Several other smaller photos in a stack showed Olive or the older woman in various vacation activities: at the beach, hiking through a jungle, standing at the roadside by a sign that had something written in Hawaiian. The sky was very blue in all the pictures. It looked sunny and warm.

"Umbrella drinks," I said. "Looks like you had a great time."

"It was beautiful. The weather was perfect. There is always a breeze so you don't get too hot. On the volcano we needed our jackets. It got cold up there!" Olive smiled as she looked at the photographs in my hand.

"Thanks for bringing these in for me to see." I gave the pictures back to her and stood up. "So I'll give Dr. Resh a call after you see him."

Olive wheeled herself around and I held the door open for her. "You're pretty good at that, Olive."

"Well, you know Mick is in a wheelchair so I know how they work."

"Yes, of course. I forgot about that." Olive lived with a man who needed a wheelchair as a result of a gunshot wound many years ago. I had never actually met him but he sounded like an upstanding guy. Olive had told me that he worked somewhere in the city and often traveled with her on her cruises. He did not have HIV and seemed little affected by his disability. They had a van that was modified with hand equipment so that he could drive.

Olive wheeled off down the hall and as I watched her from my office door, I saw Zoe Prin coming down the hall toward me. Zoe has a characteristic gait that comes from scoliosis. She walks with her shoulders back and always looks slightly unsteady. She passed Olive going in the other direction and as she reached me she looked over her shoulder to make sure that Olive would not overhear us. "Susan, you didn't order a CT scan, did you?"

"No, not yet. Why? Do you think she needs one?"

"No, not at all. This is totally a conversion reaction."

"What do you mean?"

"For one thing, Olive and her mother haven't seen each other for over eleven years so this trip together was really a very big deal. Then, apparently the mother unloaded a ton of old baggage on Olive, some of which she'd known about and some of which she'd never heard before. It totally overwhelmed her."

"And this is her way of dealing with it?" I asked.

"She finds comfort in the sick role. It's an escape for her."

"Well, I couldn't really find anything wrong. She's seeing the neurologist this afternoon. I was going to call him."

"I'm sure he'll tell you that your exam was correct. She's just hiding out in the wheelchair for a while because the stuff with her mom was so painful for her."

"Does she get it? That there's nothing physically wrong?"

"I didn't push her on it. Her life has been pretty terrible. I knew some of it from earlier conversations with her; she's had a lot of abuse. A stepfather who raped her when she was fourteen, a cousin who raped her when she was fifteen—very nasty. And then the mother told her about some other gruesome family episodes including a cousin who was the sex slave of a white man. It just goes on and on."

"Ay yi yi, that is grim." I didn't doubt what Zoe told me. I resolved to try to offer Olive support and not to confront her about the current need for a wheelchair.

"Terrible," agreed Zoe.

We walked together down the hall to the conference room.

In rounds that day Stan reported on a patient who had started on a combination of the medications DDI and AZT. His T cells had risen about 50 points, which Stan found encouraging. Jean then added that she'd been talking to the patient in the lab and discovered that he'd once been a good friend of Mac. There were several sighs and "oh yeahs" around the room. Mac with the long, beautiful fingers and the egg in his teeth; he'd been dead for at least two years. Several of us remembered him with great fondness. Jean said that the friend, Stan's patient, still had some of Mac's clothes and from time to time he and other friends put the clothes on and had a cocktail in honor of Mac. It sounded a bit macabre but it probably would have made Mac smile.

When Olive's name came up, Zoe and I both talked about her inability to walk. Zoe gave a brief synopsis of her meeting with Olive and her sense that this was a conversion reaction as opposed to a neurological problem.

Mikla was not Olive's social worker but she spoke up. "I saw Olive get out of a van in the hospital driveway today. There was a guy driving the van. She got out on the passenger side and went around to the back and opened the hatch door and pulled out a wheelchair. She unfolded the wheelchair and pushed it up onto the sidewalk and then sat down in the wheelchair and wheeled herself up to the hospital entrance."

Stan hooted with laughter. Gerald smiled and ran his hand through his hair. I had to laugh too and shook my head. You just can't make this stuff up, I thought. Zoe nodded her head with a satisfied look on her face. I felt glad that we weren't going to launch into a big workup for Olive's inability to walk. It seemed quite clear that she could walk if she needed to.

I thought about Olive later as I got my coat and shut off my computer for the day. As outrageous as the story seemed—that she could get the wheelchair out of the van and plop herself down in it—the underlying reason for Olive's behavior was almost ungraspable in its sadness. We could laugh about it perhaps only because it was too late to cry. And Olive had made her way forward as best she could out of her awful circumstances. She lived with a guy who seemed steady and decent; she had never bailed out into heroin or crack. Hell, she went on more cruises than anyone I ever knew! Yes, vast amounts of time and resources had been spent on Olive over the years; we had often judged her because of it. Today she needed to roll around in a wheelchair to get past some demons. You could say it deviated a bit from ordinary coping mechanisms, such as sweaty workout sessions or multiple martinis. For Olive the wheelchair was a safe and protected place where she could rest for a while.

What kind of woman was her mother? There she stood in the photo with Olive, holding her umbrella drink and smiling under the palm tree, no indication of Olive's trauma in either of their faces. Had she known about what Olive was going through? Had she tried to protect her daughter? And what about Pat with her sixteen-year-old? What kind of mother could she possibly be? Would that sixteen-year-old ever stand on a beach with her arm around Pat and smile into the camera? And me? What kind of mother would I be? These were exhausting questions, none with easy answers. Or maybe I was exhausted because I was twenty-eight weeks pregnant and working full-time.

# Chapter Ten

# 1995 Decisions and Revisions

Etta came for an appointment one morning very late in my pregnancy. I'd still been unable to get her to accept any prescriptions from me. We all worried what would happen to her little son, Joey, if she should ever get sick and need to be in the hospital. That time must surely be coming, I thought. Her T cells continued to decline and her immune system grew steadily weaker. She'd been heavyset when I first met her, fussed up with her pink lipstick and finely plucked eyebrows. Now she looked exhausted and pale, her hair rough and dull; she'd lost weight. After walking slowly into my office with me, she sat down panting in the chair.

"Well, I did what you said." She spoke between breaths.

"What do you mean?" I asked, sitting down across the desk.

"I took that stuff."

"You mean the Bactrim?"

"Is that the big white pill?"

"Usually, yeah, it's pretty big."

"No, no," she said, shaking her head and waving her hand as if to shoo away a bad smell. "That pill was way too big."

"What stuff then? What did I give you?"

"That AZT. But it didn't work."

"I gave you AZT?" I started hunting around in her chart for the notes from previous visits. I didn't think I had put her on AZT recently but maybe I just didn't remember.

"You did, somebody did. I can't remember. The bottle was from a while ago." Etta spoke in a bored voice. Despite looking sick, she still had her aloof and can't-be-bothered attitude.

I looked up from her chart. When I first met her two years ago, she told me she'd been given AZT in the past but took it for only a month or so. "You were given AZT when you were at East General."

"Yeah. I had the bottle still so I started taking it again. But I don't feel any better. You know, I'm losing weight and I can't eat too good and my hair is falling out. The AZT didn't help. That stuff doesn't work. Now I feel even worse."

"How long have you been taking AZT? How much did you take?"

"Well, the bottle says five times a day so I was taking three or four pills. Five seemed too many."

"And when did you start doing this?"

"About a month ago or so. I went back to the pharmacist to get some more but he said I should call you since the prescription was old. But it wasn't working anyway so I just stopped." She started looking at her long pink-lacquered fingernails.

"Etta, why didn't you call us?"

"What for?"

"Well, if you were feeling bad, I would like to know that. Your social worker, the nurses. That's what we're here for. We want to know how you're doing. And I need to know if you're taking medications that I didn't give you."

"Don't worry, I won't be taking any more of it. Those pills gave me such a headache."

AZT often did give people headaches at first so I didn't doubt that she'd been taking it. But AZT could also cause significant anemia. That might be why Etta looked so pale.

"Are you short of breath?"

"Yeah, carrying Joey up the stairs I need to stop. He has to walk up himself."

"And then you walk up too?"

"No, I rest. I give him the keys to get in and after a while I can go up."

"Are you coughing?"

"No, not really. I just can't eat, though."

"When did you stop taking the AZT?"

"Probably a week ago. I've been in bed for about a week."

Her story felt to me like verbal quicksand. Every new piece of information made things sound worse and the chaos rattled me. Taking a deep breath I said, "OK, Etta, let's start again." Maybe if I made a coherent story I could feel as if I had some control. "You were home feeling bad and a month ago you started taking some old AZT that you had. You took it three or four times a day for a month or so. In that time you didn't feel better but began feeling more and more tired. Last week you stopped the AZT and have been in bed at home since then."

"Yeah," she said, looking at the ceiling as if I'd just recited a long poem in Urdu. "Can I lie down for a little while?"

"Certainly. Have you been in bed because you've been tired? Or is there something else that's been wrong to make you want to lie down? Fevers, chest pain, dizziness, anything?"

"Well, Joey was at his grandmother's so he was out of my hair and I just felt tired."

"Did you have fever?"

"No. But I did get dizzy sometimes."

"Let me examine you and we can send off some blood tests to find out what's going on. I think you should stay in the hospital, though."

She got up from her chair and sat on the examining table where the white paper seemed to match the color of her face. That brief effort left her panting again; she nodded yes when I asked if she felt dizzy. Her heart beat fast and thin like a bird's. The conjunctiva around her eyes, even the inside of her mouth looked pale. I had her lie down and then sit up, checking her pulse and blood pressure. Her pressure dropped and her heart rate sped up and again she felt dizzy with the change in position. Everything told me her blood count was low but the important question was why. I found no evidence of bleeding, so either the red cells were being destroyed or she wasn't making enough. I suspected the AZT had worsened anemia brought on by her profound immune deficiency. She walked with me slowly down the hall to one of the other examining rooms where she could lie down for a bit. Midway down the hall she said, "I'm thinking about getting pregnant in the spring."

I thought I might have misheard her. Maybe she'd said, "I'm drinking something stagnant in a string." No. That wasn't it.

"Etta," I said, "let's see what's happening with you now. Let's get you better first, OK?"

"Yeah." She could hardly say more, it took so much effort.

"Does seeing me make you think of it?"

"Yeah," she said again. She got onto the examining table and lay back with her eyes closed. I stood looking at her for a while, watching the little blue vein pulsate in the side of her neck. I wished we had something more comfortable for her to lie on. Just then I felt the baby inside me squirm and wiggle. God, I felt lucky. And guilty. I had a sensation of enormous relief that it wasn't me lying there on that table. Etta looked so weak and tired. How could she possibly be thinking of having a baby when she was having a very hard time just getting down the hall? Perhaps it helped her to imagine a future of possibilities and new life. I realized that beneath my white coat and stethoscope I existed in that quasi-stupor of first pregnancy, almost like a narcotic in its self-indulgence. I couldn't blame her for wanting to feel that way.

Most patients hadn't noticed my pregnancy until recently. Now it seemed that people enjoyed the distraction of asking me questions instead of answering mine. How was I feeling? Was I having a boy or a girl? Did I have any names picked out? When would I come back to work?

I had this vague sense of being with someone during my pregnancy and it unexpectedly made my patients seem more alone. Once, on a weekend on call, I rounded on a patient of Maggie's who had come in with pneumonia and diffuse joint pains. I stood next to the man's bed and asked him how he was feeling. Although his chart indicated that he was improving steadily, he complained of feeling terrible. A fairly stocky guy in his mid-sixties with a bushy gray mustache, he spoke bitterly of how AIDS had ruined his life. Unable to face the sympathy or fear that he saw in the eyes of his family and friends, he had completely isolated himself and felt utterly lonely and bitter. He talked and talked; he didn't ask me for anything and he didn't seem to want anything from me but an occasional nod of my head. As I listened to him the baby inside me rolled over and kicked. This sensation usually made me smile or chuckle, or at the very least rub the spot on my protruding belly. But standing there listening to the patient's litany of problems, I didn't feel that I could smile or chuckle or draw attention to any aspect of myself. The man needed so badly to have someone simply be with him and hear him, to have someone pay undivided attention, if only for a few moments. He talked about his medications, his aches and pains, his intravenous line, his difficulty breathing. He talked about the nurses waking him in the middle of the night to take his temperature, then leaving him staring at the ceiling, unable to find his way back into sleep. Eventually I asked him if I could sit down and he seemed glad to say yes. I think I spent only ten minutes or so sitting on his bed listening and nodding while the baby who would be my son Jules kicked and waved around inside me. After a while I got up to continue seeing the other patients on my rounds. I thanked the patient for allowing me to stop and rest for a while. He said he was glad to have helped and he appreciated my being there to talk to. As I left his room I felt acutely aware of the company I carried with me; I looked back to see the patient sitting alone in his hospital bed holding the television remote. I thought again of this man as I looked at Etta lying on the stretcher with her eyes closed.

Jean went in to draw Etta's blood and send it to the lab. Within an hour the blood test returned, showing severe anemia. We couldn't do transfusions in the clinic and there was no way I was sending her home. I called the resident to arrange for her admission to the hospital. The escort came up with a wheelchair to take Etta down to the emergency room so that she could get a blood transfusion.

At lunchtime a little later I went to the floor to see Luz. Her untreatable hepatitis had caused her liver to fail and her abdomen swelled with fluid on a regular basis. The last year and a half had seen a slow but steady deterioration. She'd been admitted at two a.m. the night before for the fourth time in as many months. The house staff were starting to call her my frequent flyer, a term that I understood but didn't care for. Once she was up in a bed in the hospital, the admitting team had removed over a gallon of fluid from her abdomen. She seemed to be sleeping soundly when I knocked softly on her door and walked in. Even under the sheets and blankets I could see her huge abdomen. I spoke her name softly and her small, dark sunken eyes opened in a face that looked thin and sickly yellow.

"Hey," I said quietly to her.

"Hi, Dr. Ball."

"How are you?"

"Not so good, I guess."

"Do you have pain?"

She shifted a little in the bed. Her abdomen shifted with her like a large bale of something beneath the covers. "No, I don't have pain. I just can't move very good."

"Have you had any fever?" Fever for Luz might mean the fluid was infected, which could be a catastrophe. Every time we put a needle into her abdomen to drain the fluid we risked infection. It felt like the odds against her worsened every day.

"No, I don't think I had fever. Just hard to move. I'm sorry to come back so soon."

"Oh brother, Luz, please don't apologize. I'm glad you got a bed. Remember two weeks ago when you were stuck in the ER for nearly three days?"

She smiled weakly at that. Her hair had thinned, dark wavy hair that fell over her face. The last admission had been a nightmare for her. Not that the nightmare had ended.

"How's Toby?"

"He's good. He's at my sister's."

"Is it OK if I sit down?" I moved her bedside table so that I could sit on the end of her bed. "Do you feel better this morning since they took off the fluid?"

"I feel a little better."

"You are still pretty tight, aren't you?" I said, patting the covers over her abdomen. I felt no give, no shift. No jiggle indicating fluid inside.

"They said they'd take some more off today. They didn't want to do too much in the middle of the night."

"Yeah, I think that was a good idea. We'll check your labs again this morning, too."

"It came back fast this time." She looked at me questioningly.

I nodded, looking at her. We had talked before of Luz's thoughts about the future. Her prognosis contained no relief and we both knew this situation would continue to worsen. Liver transplant might be an option for another patient, someone who could get on the list and go to Pittsburgh to wait for months or years. Luz had HIV and no one would put her on a transplant list. Two fatal illnesses. Her family knew only about the hepatitis. She had never told them about the HIV. She worried they would reject her, not help with Toby, never come and see her. I thought they should know but I didn't push her to tell them. HIV seemed the least of her problems these days. She'd never had any symptoms of HIV, not even thrush. She had a good T cell count and I didn't have her on any medication. It would be a few more years before we understood that co-infection with HIV led to more rapid progression of the chronic liver disease caused by Hepatitis C.

I sighed. Luz was right. The fluid had reaccumulated within two weeks. Previously she'd had at least a month between admissions. The circle of her downward spiral was closing. I had a foreboding image of being too far inside a cave at the beach as the tide is coming in. "You know, we talked about surgery. About a shunt," I said to her.

"I know. You said it wouldn't work."

Had I really said it wouldn't work? It made me wince to think that that was the message she had taken away from our conversation of a few weeks ago. A shunt would be a way to give her abdomen a little relief by pulling off some of the fluid and putting it back into her circulation. Unfortunately, shunts were notoriously dangerous and complicated. Her HIV scared the surgeons as well. A shunt could be offered until something better came along, but in Luz's case something better didn't exist. I didn't want to give her false hope by telling her about a treatment option that wouldn't really help, but I felt she needed to know about the procedure.

"Luz," I said, "I think that a shunt would probably relieve some of this pressure in your belly. It won't cure the hepatitis or help your liver. The procedure itself is not that hard, but all the fluid shifting around can cause a lot of problems. It's not been shown yet to really make much of a difference for people."

"It doesn't work."

I smiled at her with a heavy feeling in my chest. No bullshit. She saw right through me. "I'm trying to be honest with you. But I think maybe you are being more honest than I am."

I wanted to offer her some kind of alternative to this awful course. I must have been talking just to hear my own voice because I was not fooling Luz. When you put your ear on the railroad tracks you can hear the train far off. I recognized the sounds on the rails and wished I had something more to offer her while inside I was shaking my fists at my powerlessness.

Luz sighed. A tear rolled down the side of her cheek. "So what happens now?"

"Well, we've talked before. It's never the right time and I don't think that this is going to happen right now, but you said that you didn't want to be on a breathing machine. Do you still feel that way?"

"No machines. This is bad enough, Toby seeing me like this."

"I don't think you need a breathing machine at all at this point. But I need to ask you about it each time you come into the hospital. I worry that you are getting a little more fragile each time I see you."

"Yeah," she said and reached her hand out from under the covers for a tissue on the table by her bed. "How's my T cells?"

"Your T cells are fine. The last time we checked I think there were four hundred and fifty or something close to that."

"Four hundred and sixty-two."

"There you go. We haven't done them yet on this admission. It's not likely they will have changed much at all. Your HIV, fortunately, is not a problem."

"How soon can I go home?"

"Well, soon I hope, but let's see how today goes. I want the GI people to come back and see you. We need to make you more comfortable but as you can see, the fluid is coming back each time a little faster."

"I just couldn't wait anymore, I couldn't breathe."

"No, I know, it's terrible for you. The problem is that your albumin level gets lower and lower partially because you lose some each time we take off these large amounts of fluid. Your liver isn't making any new albumin in the way that it should. Albumin helps hold fluid in the bloodstream. Without it the liquid, the water in the circulation, seeps out into your abdomen. That's a rough way of describing what is happening."

"Can't I just get more albumin?"

"It doesn't last for very long but we do that sometimes. That's what I want to ask the GI doctors about. It's not a long-term answer but it might help a little for a while." I didn't want to tell Luz that we'd tried this several times with her in the past and though it had been transiently beneficial, it almost seemed to accelerate the overall deterioration.

I spent a few more minutes with Luz, examining her heart and lungs, looking at her legs to see if there was extra fluid there as well. The palms of her hands were red and she had little broken blood vessels in various places on the surface of her skin, all signs of her cirrhosis. I left her room and hoped she'd at least find some relief in going back to sleep.

Stan sat at the nurses' station writing notes. He'd been going back and forth to Virginia for several months and in the last few weeks his mother had finished her chemotherapy and seemed to be doing quite well. "Good morning, Dr. Singular," he said, looking up. He was referring to my slightly demented patient William, who had called me Dr. Balls just yesterday. When I'd corrected William by telling him it's singular, he promptly called me Dr. Singular.

"Don't worry. He called me Dr. Balls again this morning."

Stan chuckled and went back to his writing. I pulled out Luz's chart and sat down next to him to read the notes from the admission.

Maureen, one of the nurses, came in. "Oh my God," she said to Stan. "I can't believe that."

Stan looked up at her and laughed.

"What happened?" I asked.

"Georgina's eye," said Maureen.

"Georgina P.," said Stan. "She's had a glass eye for years from some trauma when she was young. Now, though, she's lost so much weight that the eye doesn't fit very well. It falls out."

"I was talking to her and she sneezed and her eye popped out and landed on the floor!" added Maureen.

"Oh my God."

"It rolled under the radiator. She told me to rinse it off in the sink and give it back to her. And she just popped it right back in!"

Stan leaned back in his chair smiling and shaking his head as he listened to Maureen tell this story. Maureen gave another chuckle and picked up her medication book. "I wonder how many more times that's going to happen today," she said, walking out of the nurses' station and heading down the hall.

I looked at Stan.

He looked back at me and shook his head again. "Fuckin' A," he said. Then he returned to writing his notes and I returned to Luz's chart. After reading the residents' notes I wrote my own and then went down the hall to see my next patient.

I knocked on the door and Marco's mother said, come in. The window in the room looked out over an interior courtyard. Most of the room was in shadow but for a dim light over the empty hospital bed. Marco's mother sat in the half-lit space near the window.

"Hello, Mrs. Prava."

"Hello, Dr. Ball." She always greeted me in a way that seemed quite formal, but over the last few weeks I had come to know her as warm and articulate.

"Where's Marco?"

"He's gone to have an X-ray"

"Has he been gone a long time?"

"Not that long, maybe twenty minutes."

"You're sitting here in the dark."

"Yes. I'm waiting for him to come back."

"How is he today?" I went closer and sat on the ledge of the window facing her.

"He's about the same. Very weak."

"Very weak." I sat looking at her in the gloomy room. The vaguely foul odor of disinfectant over feces wafted about us. There had been times when this room defied the strongest stomach because of the smell. Today wasn't bad. *Cryptosporidium*, the infection in Marco's colon, caused a constant watery diarrhea. Day and night it had slowly sapped all his strength, all his fat, all his muscle mass. No known effective cure existed for *Cryptosporidium* and it seemed that nothing we gave him helped the diarrhea. Marco's body epitomized the expression "skin and bones." On the bedside table stood a photograph of Marco and his mother in another time and place. They smiled together looking at the camera while palm trees waved in the background. The tall, handsome man in the photograph had brown eyes and broad shoulders and looked nothing like the Marco I saw suffering and wasting away each day in this miserable hospital bed.

Soon we'd be deciding whether Marco should go home in his mother's care or to a nursing home. Although I'd discussed the options with both of them a couple of times, they were not considering anything other than Marco going home with his mother. I wanted to offer an alternative. Having him at home was going to be a tremendous strain on them both. We could help by setting up nursing services and a home attendant for support with changing beds and doing laundry. But Marco needed constant care and he and I both worried about how this would affect his mother.

I looked at Marco's empty bed, with its clean sheets stretched tightly across and a knitted blue blanket from home folded at the foot. "Mrs. Prava, how are you doing?"

"I'm all right," she said. Funny, I thought to myself. Someone I know said just the same thing a long time ago.

"Are you getting enough rest?"

"I get home late but I guess I do, yes."

"Marco told you to stop sleeping here, didn't he?"

"Marco is worried about me." She gave a little chuckle, looking at the floor. "Marco, worrying about his mama."

I waited for her to say more.

She lifted her head and looked right at me. "He has the AIDS, doesn't he?"

Her question surprised me. I had assumed that she knew. But in fact I had never actually spoken to her about it. The diarrhea came from an infection that we spoke of very freely, but AIDS had opened the door for that infection. We had never overtly discussed the underlying cause. Too many assumptions. I felt my face turn red.

"Mrs. Prava, I . . ."

"I have known for a long time. You don't need to worry about telling me. Marco did not want me to worry. He wants to protect me." She was looking past me, talking more to herself. "I have known for a long time that Marco has the AIDS. He might even think now that I don't know. We don't talk about it anymore. We are just trying to take care of him. To get him to eat a little bit. The diarrhea; it is so strong.

"Before, when he was better, he had a friend who came to our house a lot. A beautiful young man, so handsome and so funny. Always sweet to me and a good friend for Marco. And then he was not coming to our house so much and when he came I asked Marco, what is wrong with Eric? He is so thin and his pants are falling down from his hips. Marco said he didn't know. And then Eric came one last time and he was coughing and sweating and he cried when he said good-bye. I said to Marco, this boy has the AIDS and he is dying, and Marco said, 'No, Mommy, he is just sick. He is OK. He will get better, don't worry.' But I knew that that boy was sick with the AIDS. And then Marco started to not eat well and he was swimming in his shirts and wearing his belt four holes tighter. I have known for a long time. I am his mother and I will take care of him."

She wasn't looking at me and her voice quavered a little as she talked, holding a crumpled tissue in her hand. A thin gold wedding band looked tight on her finger and I imagined the young girl she must have been when it was first placed there. Now she was a bit heavyset; she wore glasses with metal frames and a simple flowered dress and tan shoes with low heels. The dark wool coat that she'd taken off and folded on the back of the chair didn't look warm enough. She brushed at something on her lap and balled the tissue into her fist. She didn't cry.

"Mrs. Prava, I think that Marco worries about you nearly as much as you worry about him."

She gave a little shake of her head saying, "Marco."

"I know we have been over this and I think everyone wants Marco to be able to come home and stay."

"It's really the only place for him."

"I know, you're right," I continued. "But there is so much care that he needs. I worry about both of you."

"I can't send him to a nursing home."

"I know. I know you can't. We're going to try to make this work. I just, well, I just feel a bit worried that it will be too hard." I knew that I could bulldoze this situation and send Marco to a nursing home. He might get better professional care there. But really Marco needed his mother and the love she brought him. She'd end up practically living at the nursing home anyway. I thought again about listening to the distant vibration of the railroad tracks.

The only power I had in this situation was to help Marco die peacefully in his home with his mother near him.

"Dr. Ball, you are very kind."

"Mrs. Prava, what you are doing for Marco is so important and so wonderful. Many patients here are alone. Marco is lucky."

She hesitated for a moment. "No. Marco is not lucky."

God, had I really said that? Marco is lucky? Shitting on himself within minutes of having the last soiled diaper changed? Wracked by cramps and smelling either of feces or that horrible peppermint air freshener that sits like glue in the air? Unable to walk or dress or laugh or read or even have a conversation? Lucky?

"I'm sorry. I said the wrong thing. What I want to say is that Marco has something that so many people with this illness lack. He has someone who loves him. He is here in a great hospital and I don't think that he'd get better care anywhere else, but the most important thing is your love and your presence. That's what I meant to say."

"It's all right. I know what you meant."

"I wish there was more that we could do to help."

"It will be good to go home."

I got up and reached out to touch her hand. She looked down at her lap. My beeper went off and I fumbled with it to make it stop. Then I put my hand on Mrs. Prava's shoulder. "I'll see you later," I said, and went to the door.

The resident in the emergency room had paged me to tell me that Etta was trying to leave. They were still waiting for the blood to come up from the lab. As we spoke the resident in the ER said Etta was standing next to him and had agreed to talk to me before she left. He handed the phone over to her.

"Etta," I said, "why are you going home? Please stay in the hospital. I'm really worried about you. You really need to get a blood transfusion."

"I can come back tomorrow. I have some things to do at home." I could hear all the random voices and beeping of the busy emergency room in the background.

"Why didn't you say anything before? Why do you have to go now?"

"I'll be back tomorrow. I just have to do some things."

"I don't get it." I heard myself practically pleading with her. "You're really sick. You need to be in the hospital. Joey's at your mother's. What is it that's so important to do at home?"

"Well, I have some laundry that I have to do." She sounded thoroughly irritated with me.

"Laundry?"

"I'll call you tomorrow. I'll be OK. My father is coming to pick me up."

I couldn't believe what I was hearing. "Etta, I can't force you to stay but I really think it's important for you to be in the hospital."

"Here, the doctor wants to talk to you." Somehow I could picture Etta rolling her eyes at my nagging voice.

The resident came back on the phone. "Dr. Ball, she has her coat on and everything. What do you want us to do?"

"She's an adult," I said, more to myself than to him. "Of course I don't agree with her decision but we can't force her to stay. It's just, it's just . . . Will you tell her to eat some steak or spinach or something tonight?" I actually laughed as I said this; images of Popeye gulping down a can of spinach and *poof*, there would be muscles and strength.

The resident chuckled, as if he'd seen the same image. "Yeah, sure."

"And please make her sign an AMA form. I wish she wouldn't do this."

"It's been a wild day down here," he said. "I'll get her to sign the form."

I hung up the phone and stood at the nurses' station looking at the bulletin board by the clerk's desk. She had to go home and do her laundry. What did that mean? The emergency room could be the most unfriendly, noisy, uncomfortable place to be. Who wouldn't rather be home? Then I thought of what she'd said to me walking down the hall. She's thinking about having a baby. What could I tell her? Don't have a baby? You have a fatal illness, you don't take care of yourself, and your unborn child stands a thirty percent chance of also being infected? You are going to leave your children without a mother? All these things went through my mind. I felt like a hypocrite being pregnant and thinking that pregnancy should be strictly avoided by someone like Etta. What did I know? And who was I to judge? I thought of Marco's mother sitting there in the dimly lit room, and of Luz with her belly full of fluid. Goddammit, Etta was thinking of getting pregnant next spring. In the meantime she was going home to do her goddamn laundry.

# Chapter Eleven

# 1995  Colleagues and Families

Sabitha had a smile that rivaled that of my old patient Mac: you just couldn't help but smile back. When she first came to the hospital with PCP in 1994, she did not look like a twenty-four-year-old mother of four; she looked like a nubile young teenager. Lustrous hair set off dimples and sparkling dark eyes. Her dead ex-boyfriend, the father of the three younger kids, had never told her about his AIDS diagnosis. Miraculously, none of the kids carried the virus. Sabitha seemed strangely apathetic when I talked with her of the diagnosis of PCP, which meant she had AIDS, as if the information had stopped on the doorstep of her brain but not entered. I tried to imagine what she must be feeling: dead boyfriend, four children, AIDS; who could imagine being in that life?

She'd had an uncomplicated hospital course and the PCP responded well to the treatment. Once discharged from the hospital, though, she missed many of her CSS appointments. Four kids is a lot of kids. I gained new appreciation for this, as my son Jules was born the year after I first met Sabitha. One child at home created an entirely new dimension of obligations and responsibilities. The thought of four children made me slightly dizzy. A year after her first admission Sabitha came back into the hospital.

I stood in the hospital room with her, trying to figure out why she was talking so oddly and why her muscles seemed to be losing their strength. Admitted from home after two months of progressive weakness, she had muscle spasticity and her legs would not hold her up. She could move them and could move her arms as well, but her muscles jerked uncontrollably at times and she spilled her food when she tried to eat. She complained that her left leg felt numb and that her hands would jerk suddenly on their own. She'd also had a gradual change in her voice that caused her to speak in a nasal, halting way. When I asked her why she hadn't called me when this started two months ago, she told me that she'd been frightened; she didn't want to get bad news. Her fears were justified; things did not look good. The neurologists shook their heads and shrugged their shoulders. We waited to see the brain images from the CT scan.

In the area of the cerebrum where the scan should be gray and uniformly colored, we saw instead a lot of large white cotton ball–type abnormalities. The brain itself was smaller than it should be for a woman her age. On scan, Sabitha's brain looked like a big old shriveled prune.

So now Sabitha, at twenty-five years old, had what radiographically looked like the brain of a ninety-year-old. Her appearance had changed markedly as well. Coarse, lumpy skin and dull, dry hair took the place of her previously dewy complexion and thick, shining mane. All the muscle twitches and spasticity and the abnormal CT scan led us to give her a diagnosis of AIDS encephalopathy or possibly something called progressive multifocal leukoencephalopathy (PML). Both resulted from advanced immune suppression and affected the central nervous system. A biopsy might differentiate between the two, but it didn't matter which of these she had as no treatment existed for either one. The likelihood of recovery seemed all but nonexistent, and although she took two drugs for her HIV, her T cells remained very low. We talked to her about going to a nursing home but she insisted on going home to be with her children. I knew that her being at home could not last long; soon Sabitha would need more care than we could provide for her as an outpatient.

Sabitha's current boyfriend came to the hospital to bring her home. He gently helped her to get out of bed and get dressed. With his dark crew cut, gray hooded sweatshirt, diamond earring, and black baseball hat he looked barely twenty years old. As he pushed her wheelchair down the hall, Sabitha didn't look up or wave good-bye. She seemed so tiny, her little hands holding the armrests, sitting there engulfed in her big green down parka.

I took it as a good sign that the boyfriend had pulled me aside one afternoon to ask about the effectiveness of condoms for protection against transmission of HIV. He told me he'd tested negative for HIV and he wanted to know about the medication for Sabitha, whether it could help her, whether it could work. In the previous year she had taken AZT and another anti-HIV medication called lamivudine, but her T cells had not budged. She was going home on a combination of still two more medicines, but I told him honestly that I didn't anticipate much improvement with this regimen either. The list of future options to treat the virus remained very short; all approved medications consisted of variations on the mechanism of AZT. We looked at each other with frustration. Sabitha's future appeared grim.

I had heard some exciting rumors of new drugs now under study. We had several patients already participating in various clinical trials with medications that interrupted different aspects of the replication cycle of HIV. The drugs had not yet been approved by the FDA so they remained unavailable, but we sensed a buzz of excitement about the possibilities. I likened our position to being in a sniper battle against a huge and powerful enemy, dodging through the bushes, not sure where you are, wanting to believe that help is coming but not knowing when it will get here or how effective it will be if it ever does. I told Sabitha's boyfriend that we all hoped the new medications would be better than what we had now, that with luck they'd come soon. He looked at me searchingly and then shook his head, saying, "It's not like she's the only one, huh?" I watched them leave the hospital floor that day, going home to four young children. Children going home to children; old before their time, dying before their time.

When her name came up during inpatient rounds the next day, I reported that Sabitha had already been discharged. Sister Harriet asked how she'd gotten home and Molly, Sabitha's social worker, said the boyfriend had been amazingly helpful and supportive. He had taken her home and was helping with the kids, getting them to school. "He's a pretty remarkable guy," said Molly. "I don't know how long he's going to last with this situation. Sabitha has become so helpless and her mother is a bad alcoholic. The four kids are pretty wild."

"Is the boyfriend positive?" Dr. Jacobs asked.

"He told me that he's negative," I said, "and I think he's pretty reliable. He seems like a good guy."

"Let's talk about inpatients who are still here," said Gerald. "Who's next?" he asked, looking toward Pam, the nurse sitting there with her medication book.

"Next is Dierdre G."

Stan, by the window next to me, leaned his chair back against the wall and sighed. A few people smiled. "Dierdre's here with back pain. She has six hundred T cells and I think the back pain is just muscular but I admitted her to try to expedite the MRI and get neurosurgery to see her. It's a bit soft for an admit but she was driving me crazy with phone calls for pain meds."

"Some doctor you are," said Dr. Jacobs.

"She said her foot was numb!" Stan protested, sitting forward again.

"And you believed it?"

I thought of Dierdre doing the Macarena at the Christmas party. How Stan had mimed weighing the options in his hands, suicide or Macarena.

"Nursing," interrupted Gerald. He wanted to keep us on track and he looked expectantly at Pam. She looked down at her medication book.

"Dierdre's been ambulating in the hall and asking to go downstairs to smoke. This morning she's afebrile. Her blood pressure's fine. She's been getting oxycodone around the clock, which she says has been helpful for her back pain. She's written for it every four hours."

"Has neurosurgery seen her?" asked Stan.

"The house staff called the consult but I don't think they've come yet."

Briana, the social worker on the case, spoke up. "Dierdre's a thirty-seven-year-old woman who was diagnosed in 1990. Her risk factor is unprotected heterosexual contact. She's divorced with no children and has an apartment in Queens. Her boyfriend moved in a few weeks ago. She has Medicaid, Medicare, food stamps, and HASA benefits." Lots of our patients got financial aid from HASA, the city's HIV/AIDS Services Administration. "She says the boyfriend will give her a ride home when she's discharged."

"Sounds like our patients have very supportive boyfriends," observed Dr. Jacobs.

"Well, yesterday Dierdre told me that her supportive boyfriend is wanted for murder," said Stan.

There were gasps around the room and Dr. Jacobs's mouth dropped open. Stan smiled and he shrugged his shoulders. "She says he's a great guy and he's very nice to her. What can I say?"

"How about the word 'criminal'?"

Gerald, ever mindful, spoke up, "Aren't you obligated to call the police? Get his name?"

"She says he didn't do it, he was in another part of the city when it happened."

"Oh, like Son of Sam?"

"Well, I believe her but that doesn't mean I believe *him*!"

"I met him," Briana chimed in. "He had very nice aftershave."

"Those were the murder victim's last words," said Dr. Jacobs, rolling his eyes.

"Wait, wait," said Dr. Berry. "What Dierdre told me is that her boyfriend was supposed to go in to talk to the police about some murder case that happened a few years ago. He was involved somehow with the victim but he isn't a suspect."

"How convenient."

"No, I really think it's fine. Dierdre's choice in men is not stellar historically but I don't think she's in danger or sheltering a criminal or anything like that."

"That is a huge relief," said Gerald. "We could have been accessories."

"Or worse," added Dr. Jacobs.

"Well that's disappointing," said Stan.

"You mean that he's not a murderer?" asked Gerald.

"Go ahead, say it. You were hoping," said Dr. Jacobs.

"She told me he was wanted for murder," Stan said, protesting but laughing.

"And you thought you'd have one less patient to take care of."

"I'm sure he's a perfectly upstanding guy."

"Who's involved in a murder case."

"And smells good."

"And is supportive."

"Next," said Gerald.

Stan tilted his chair back again and took a sip from his coffee cup. For Friday rounds we pushed all the chairs and couches against the walls in the bright solarium on our inpatient floor. With all the doctors, floor nurses, social workers, the nutritionist, physical therapist, and Sister Harriet, about twenty-five people participated in the rounds. Maggie, back from a vacation in Greece, sat across the room looking tanned and rested.

As the nurse for the next patient began speaking, Stan leaned sideways toward me and, without taking his eyes off the nurse, said in a low voice, "She's got a new boyfriend."

"Maggie?" I whispered back.

He nodded.

"From her trip?"

He nodded again.

"That's great," I said, looking over at Maggie. Good for her, I thought. We both listened as Maggie spoke after the nurse. Her patient had been admitted with a seizure and the neurosurgeons didn't want to do a brain biopsy of the lesion revealed by the brain scan.

"He's illiterate," Stan said, out of the side of his mouth.

"What?"

"He can't read or write."

Now the social worker spoke about the patient and Stan and I listened intently, not looking at each other. As Sister Harriet started to present her view of the patient, I leaned toward Stan and whispered, "The boyfriend can't read or write?"

Stan still didn't look at me but smiled and shook his head.

"Dennis P.," said Gerald, moving on to the next patient.

"Oh, poor Dennis," said Stan leaning forward so that the four legs of his chair were on the ground. "He got admitted last night. He's a forty-seven-year-old man who hasn't been to clinic for over a year but showed up yesterday looking pretty terrible. I'm not even sure how he got here since he could hardly stand up. He's lost thirty-five pounds since I last saw him. He says he can't eat. His throat was full of thrush; he's likely got esophagitis as well. He wasn't even aware of it but he's nearly blind in his left eye. Ophtho saw him last night and he has advanced CMV retinitis."

"Isn't he the guy who threw the chair through the window?" Gerald asked.

"Yeah. A few years ago. That seems unlikely this time around."

"Wow, at least he's still alive."

"It's a good thing he's getting admitted," said Suzette. "The VNS called this morning to say that his apartment is such a wreck and so disgusting that they're not going back in there. They wanted us to know that he fired his home attendant." Sometimes I thought about some of the apartments and living spaces that the visiting nurses went to. Those nurses definitely did not get paid enough money.

"Social work?" said Gerald, looking up.

"He hasn't had a home attendant in over a month." This came from Warren, Dennis's social worker. Warren often played with his pencil in his fingers when he spoke. He did so today and I saw that he had white patches under his fingernails. "His phone's been shut off so he didn't let us know, and the agency claims it was up to the patient to tell us."

"He kicked her out? How has he been getting any food?" Gerard asked.

"I don't know." He paused. Warren was a soft-spoken, sweet fellow but he occasionally drove me crazy in clinic rounds because he talked so slowly. He'd say something like "George wants new housing." And thinking about things for a moment, he'd add, "We talked about that for a while." Then, after looking at his notes for a bit, he'd say, "He has Medicaid." When rounds came after a busy clinic afternoon and we had a big pile of people to get through,

Warren's slow, deliberate approach could make me break out in a sweat. Now he continued talking about Dennis. "The agency said that he made it impossible for anyone to stay there. And they said, too, that the apartment's in horrible shape. Incredibly dirty, garbage everywhere, roaches, even rats."

Groans and ughs came from all sides of the room.

"Dennis told me that he has a neighbor who would bring him food sometimes," said Suzette.

"Well, the rats aren't a big deal for Dennis. He has a bow and arrow that he keeps in his bed." Stan smiled and took a sip from the large cup of coffee that he bought every morning from the vendor on the corner and refilled numerous times throughout the day. "When there's a rat in his room he shoots it."

"What? You are joking!" Gerald put down his pen in disbelief.

"I kid you not. That's what he told me. He even has some bow with a famous name on it that was supposed to impress me."

"Oh, come on."

"What?"

"And has he really killed a rat that way?"

"Remember, this is the guy who threw a chair through a window into the hall when his lunch was late. I don't know whether he's killed a rat or not but it sure isn't me who's going to call him a liar."

"Good point," said Gerald, looking down at his papers. "Looks like he's going to need housing." We moved on to hear about the next patient.

Eventually rounds ended, people got up to leave, and the chairs and couches were put back in their places. I walked out into the hall with Stan. "So this new squeeze of Maggie's, is he from New York?"

"No, one of the islands, some tiny place in the middle of nowhere." We were standing, waiting for the elevator to take us back upstairs.

"You mean he's Greek?"

"Nikos or Spivos or something." Stan's eyes crinkle when he's amused. He shook his head.

"You're kidding me, come on. And he can't read?" Maggie came out of the solarium just then, talking with Warren. The elevator door opened and we all joined the four or five people already on it. As we rode up to the twenty-fourth floor I looked over at Maggie as she chatted with Warren and Stan. Was she really involved with a man who couldn't read or write? Maggie prided herself on being a doctor and she took herself very seriously. She constantly read medical journals and spent a lot of time talking with the house staff and students about HIV or her patients or some other medicine-related topic. She always wore a starched white coat with her stethoscope in the pocket. Next to her I felt perpetually rumpled and wrinkled. Maggie had few activities or distractions outside of her work. An illiterate boyfriend? It seemed so unlikely, so illogical for her. But then it occurred to me that I had it all wrong. Maybe Maggie wasn't interested in having medical conversations while on her holiday. I felt a smile come over my face as I realized that perhaps this fellow had something else that he offered Maggie. A whole new side of her revealed itself to me. "La coquette!" I thought as we got to our floor and stepped off.

The reason for the white patches on Warren's fingernails became apparent over the next several weeks. I had known that he was a diabetic, but then he missed work a few times for a variety of respiratory infections. Then he missed two weeks because of pneumonia. Warren's patients noticed his absence too; he had wonderful relationships with many of them. They responded to his kindness and his quiet. Even the big, burly ex-con who swore at the front desk secretaries calmed down when Warren talked to him. With all the missed days and illness, I looked a little more closely at Warren and recognized the weight loss, the dry hair, the graying skin. Reluctantly I had to acknowledge that Warren had AIDS.

Of all places to have your AIDS diagnosis known among your co-workers, I guess CSS probably could not have been more politically correct. Everyone who knew about it—which in our case meant everyone who worked there, including the front desk secretaries and the floor janitor—wanted to help Warren in some way. His "real" HIV doctor practiced in an office downtown but everyone at CSS followed Warren's course. We wanted to know what medications he took and what allergies he had; what other illnesses he might have suffered. On the one hand, this had its benefits and I'm sure he appreciated the support and the caring. On the other hand, who really wants twenty-five caregivers watching your every move throughout the workday? We scrutinized him from across the conference table or walking down the hall: Was there any rash? Did he rub his chest? Did he look feverish? Talk about being under a microscope. Warren handled it well, but with everyone staring at him he must have felt as if he were wandering around his place of employment in boxers and socks. Of course we all asked and found out immediately that his cute boyfriend was not infected with HIV. The boyfriend worked in finance, and as Warren's HIV progressed he managed to bring Warren lunch several times a week and often dropped him off at work in the morning.

Warren worked at CSS for approximately five more months once his diagnosis was known. In that time we watched him lose weight and slow down even further in his movements and his speech. He became more fatigued. His hair thinned and he seemed less and less able to focus. To us it all happened very fast but Warren had known for years about his illness. Dr. Jacobs had known as well but it had not deterred him from hiring Warren two years prior, and Warren had worked hard and taken good care of his patients. In the late spring of 1995 he missed work for yet another illness and then did not return. The cute boyfriend stayed home with him and called Gerald from time to time with an update. Warren died that summer. Many of his patients had known of his illness and in the months that followed more than a few of them talked about Warren and their memories of him. I like to think that Warren would have appreciated the little eulogies that took place in our offices after he was gone. Years later the boyfriend gave a donation to CSS in the form of a painting of a bird on a branch. It hangs in a hallway of the hospital. Few people know that it commemorates a young man who worked hard to care for his AIDS patients and who died of the same disease.

Every spring in New York people walk all around the city for a fundraiser called the AIDS Walk. The day after the walk in 1995 the newspaper showed a picture that had been taken from the middle of the street looking at the oncoming parade. A large group of people walked toward the camera and at the head of the group a man in a white shirt held up a big sign that said BELLA.

In the hospital Bella had a room to herself. Her sister spent many nights there, keeping Bella company and sleeping in the pullout easy chair. The boys came to visit in the evenings with their uncle so I didn't often see them. Bella's husband, Cecil, came at odd times. He should have been in the hospital as well but he refused. He allowed the boys to stay with Bella's sister and brother-in-law because he couldn't care for them himself. Bella couldn't get better. Her cough got worse, she had fevers and pneumonia, she couldn't eat. The physical suffering compounded her anguish at leaving her boys and at Cecil's obvious deterioration. We stopped pressuring her to talk to Nathan, the older son, about AIDS. The situation overwhelmed all of us.

On the Monday afternoon after the AIDS Walk I sat writing notes at the nurses' station when Judy, one of the floor nurses, came up and told me that Nathan had come to visit his mother. I put my pen in my pocket and went down the hall to find him. I'd seen Nathan a couple of times in the past two years but I'd never really spoken to him; he was a shy fifteen-year-old and

I was his mother's doctor. He had never been told that Bella had AIDS. No one had sat down with him to tell him that his father and his little brother Jason had AIDS. I got to the room as he was coming out, pulling the door closed behind him. A tall, skinny kid with a few pimples and a slant of dusty brown hair over dark eyebrows, he wore huge, well-worn basketball sneakers unlaced. He looked up and, recognizing me, he stopped and put his hands in the pockets of his jeans.

"Hi, Nathan."

"Hi," he said, looking down. He didn't move.

"I don't know if you remember me. I'm Dr. Ball. I'm one of the doctors helping to take care of your mom."

He nodded but didn't say anything.

"How is your mom today?"

"She's good." He stood there looking down.

It seemed that a big cloud of noise and calamity surrounded us. I had a mouthful of things to say and a loud buzzing in my ears, like a buzz of voices shouting, "Bella is dying!" and "Bella has AIDS!" and "The boy is losing his parents!" But I just stood there, unable to think of anything to say, fumbling around in my head.

"How's Jason?" I finally managed.

"He's good."

"Your mom said you've been staying at your aunt's." We both could hear Bella coughing in her room on the other side of the door.

"Yeah." He didn't look up and still he didn't make a move to go.

"I wish," I started. I cleared my throat. "I wish that I, that there was more that we could do for your mom."

He glanced up at me ever so quickly, and I got just the briefest glimpse of hazel eyes, Bella's eyes. He looked curious and knowing, sad and empty, all at the same time. The cloud of noise around me went quiet as I watched his bent head. If there is nothing to say, it's better not to say anything. But is it? I would not lie to him and I could not tell him the truth. Is that what it is to be a doctor? Knowing that fine line between withholding details that cause pain and revealing information that is not mine to tell, even if it provides better understanding? Had he been older I would have reached out to touch his shoulder or his arm. I put my hands in the pockets of my white coat. In the right-hand pocket my hand touched a photograph of my newborn son. He's just a boy, I thought. Nathan. He's too young for this to be happening to him.

"Was it your uncle in the paper?"

He looked up again and gave an attempt at a half smile. "Yeah."

"Yeah, that was," I paused, "that was . . ." That was what? That was great? That was cool to be in the paper? That was the goddamn fundraiser so my mother doesn't fucking die of AIDS? "I thought I recognized your uncle."

"Yeah."

"Well." I reached into the breast pocket of my coat and took out one of the business cards that has my name and the clinic's number and address on it. Nowhere on the card does it say HIV or AIDS. And yet in the newspaper his uncle held a sign with his mother's name in the AIDS Walk. "Here is my card in case you might want to see me or if you have any questions. I'd be glad to talk anytime if you want to." None of us had ever betrayed Bella's privacy; none of us had ever spoken to the boys about AIDS. Still, I thought, he can't not know.

He took the card without meeting my eyes. He put his hand back into the pocket of his jeans and turned to leave. "I gotta go pick up Jason."

I watched him walk down the hall toward the elevators and Bella kept coughing in her room. I went in to see her. The view out her window looked familiar and I thought of Mr. Sullivan, the man who died in the bed where Bella now lay. I'd watched the airplanes taking off that day as I sat with him. Even now in the distance I saw an airplane lift off from the ground, just like a little staple moving up into the sky. Bella rested against her pillows with her eyes closed, the green oxygen mask covering her mouth and nose. She had purple half circles under her eyes and her long, rusty brass hair looked like a halo around her head.

"Bella?" I whispered.

"Hi, Dr. Ball," and she started coughing, sitting up and pulling the oxygen mask away from her face and reaching toward the box of tissues on her night table. I stepped over to move the tissues closer, then poured her a cup of water, which she accepted and drank before lying back and putting the mask on again.

"I just spoke to Nathan outside."

"You did?" She opened her eyes and looked at me apprehensively. I knew she wondered if I had told him about her HIV.

"I told him I'd seen your brother-in-law in the paper."

"Yeah."

No more was said. Not that day and not ten days later when Bella died in the hospital and both boys came to stand silently at her bedside while their father half-lay across her body and wept. Bella's sister and brother-in-law stood by the window, the sister quietly crying, her husband's arm around her. When they all left the boys seemed to be holding Cecil up, walking down the hall on either side of him. The sister and her husband thanked me and thanked several of the nurses on their way out. Nathan never looked at me. I would not have imagined then that I would see both boys again more than a dozen years later. But they looked awfully young on that day in 1995 when their mother died.

That year both Stan and I became parents. Stan's daughter Lizzie was born two months before my son Jules. I spent more than twelve weeks on maternity leave, a luxury almost unheard of for a doctor. Dr. Jacobs hired someone to fill in for me during my absence and this lessened the burden on my colleagues. I remember very little of that time at home with my newborn son. The first weeks seemed dreamlike as I recovered from a difficult cesarean section and we welcomed Jules into our lives. You'd think after nine months of pregnancy I would have been prepared for a baby. Hardly! I swung wildly between joy and trepidation, blissfully loving the new person in our lives and fearfully wondering how they could let us out of the hospital with this new life in our hands. My partner is an obstetrician, no novice with tiny babies. And yet the two of us were mesmerized and breathless in the face of the enormous task of caring for a newborn. People study hard and pass tests to be able to drive a car or install a toilet or practice law. It took ages of school and tests to earn a medical license. Now here we were given—without even a questionnaire!—the responsibility to care for a little baby. He utterly depended on us yet no one ever checked our qualifications. At first I cried at the slightest emotional stimulation. I cried when my mother first saw Jules and when Dr. Jacobs came to see Jules on the day he was born. I cried when we got home—"we're home!"—and when we changed Jules's diaper that first night at home with him, "his first diaper at home." And later, when I'd stopped crying all the time, I couldn't get anything done. I couldn't read or write more than a line in a thank-you note. I couldn't cook or empty the dishwasher. I nursed and changed diapers and slept and looked out the window and sometimes went for a walk with the new baby. The first time that happened I cried. "Our first walk."

I wished that Stan could have had three months off. It seemed unfair that he spent only two weeks at home when Lizzie was born. After Jules's birth I could appreciate how thoroughly life changes with a new baby. It took me all of those weeks on leave to adjust and regain my balance in order to return to work. It didn't seem right to me that Stan didn't get as much time to doze on the couch in the middle of the day with his newborn asleep on his chest, to forget he'd had breakfast because he'd been up with the baby since four thirty so he's eating chips and salsa at eight in the morning. Or to stare, speechless, for as long as he wanted, at the little grasping fingers that gripped his own, how each one had a fingernail as perfect as a Lilliputian seashell. Or even to wander around the apartment in his bathrobe until five p.m. on a Tuesday. Getting back to work didn't stop those early mornings or my staring at the fingernails, but having had more time at home made my return to work immensely less stressful, and I wished Stan could have had equal time.

Before we had babies the work at CSS had consumed our lives. But now Dr. Jacobs had two small boys, Stan had Lizzie, and I had Jules. The demands at CSS did not lessen, but our children brought us each some slight changes in perspective. Certainly our conversations broadened from mostly patient- and work-oriented to sharing our experiences at home. Lizzie didn't sleep so Stan's coffee consumption increased. Dr. Jacobs always seemed to have a vomit stain on the shoulder of his suit coat. Until I stopped nursing I pumped breast milk on an irregular schedule and often leaked through my clothes, an embarrassment I could usually hide under my white coat. We traded stories of our babies' tumults and milestones, each of us learning by trial how to do this new job of parenting.

Being a parent allowed me to appreciate another aspect of my patients' lives. We were all linked through the common experiences of friends and families, boyfriends, spouses, partners, parents, and children. The details and the stories shifted and evolved for each one of us. I could be closer to some of my patients because parenting allowed me a new perspective, a new understanding. I had a fuller appreciation for the meaning of "caregiver." I am tempted to say that being a parent helped me be a better doctor but I'm not sure that's true. Sometimes I found myself making judgments about how my patients behaved as parents. Etta referred to her little son Joey as a "pain in the ass," and Pat with the huge slice in her forehead viewed a baby as a vehicle for getting housing, not a child to bring up and care for. These attitudes shocked me. But it was like having a new window in the house: I had a different view, one to add to all the others. And being a parent no doubt changed how I looked to my patients, an added dimension to their doctor, a new window through which they could see me. I only hoped they didn't notice the soggy shirt beneath the white coat.

# Chapter Twelve

# 1995 So Many Stories and Some New Faces

Many days at CSS ended with a sense of great fatigue. I'd look at the list of people I'd seen that day and think about the stories. The tough body-builder who hated sitting with the other patients in the waiting room, the grandmother caring for five small children because her daughter was in jail, the delicate gay man with the alcoholic boyfriend, the drug addict who constantly argued for how well he could control his addiction. Story after story told to me in my office. Medicine makes a huge effort to be black and white, to find definitive answers for questions about health. What's the best way to treat a heart attack? What's the right way to set a broken bone? Where is the cancer located? Who did you get the syphilis from? When can you stop taking the blood thinner? Medicine assumes a strict objectivity, and more and more these days we have algorithms to direct our treatment decisions. And yet it is increasingly clear that there is rarely just one answer, just one treatment. It's Descartes's ultimate message, that for as much as we learn, "it is almost nothing in comparison to what remains to be discovered." AIDS humbled us. Little could be cast in black and white. No sure answers, no sure reasons. A lot of chaos in between—especially in between.

Ultimately, I can only tell *my* version, from *my* perspective. Caring for patients with HIV and AIDS, my colleagues and I learned from our experiences, but we had few definitive answers. Armed with humility we could listen to our patients, and sometimes this would be the best care of all. We could laugh to ease our pain, we could find funny the crazy, unimaginable horrors. Who could have dreamed up the woman sneezing her eyeball across the room? Our laughter was not meant to wound; on the contrary, it was a balm to soothe. I try to write things down, to be objective, but if you try to tell a story, you end up being subjective. The cold chart, in its passive voice, says, "The patient was wheeled to the operating room" or "The medication was given at six fifteen," as if these things happened without any human participation. But as patients and doctors, each of us has our own experience of events, and in trying to make sense of things, we describe what happens. If you've made it this far in my tale then you should keep going. Things got better, though not right away.

Sometime in late 1995 I met Sabir, a young man new to the clinic. When I introduced myself, he greeted me shyly and shook my hand with some hesitation. The purple mark near his hairline on the left side of his face made it obvious that Sabir had Kaposi's sarcoma. We went into my office and I learned that he was twenty-eight years old and had tested positive for HIV two years ago at an anonymous testing site. He lived in an apartment by himself down the street from his parents and sisters. They had emigrated together from Iran when Sabir was fifteen. His family did not know of his diagnosis. At first Sabir barely looked at me when he spoke and his brief answers to my questions contained only the essentials. All the while we talked his hands gripped his knees and he looked anxiously around the room. Gradually he seemed to relax a bit and he responded in longer sentences instead of one or two words.

Sabir worried that the mark on his face was like a blazing neon sign and would soon be noticed by his family. The first lesions, three or four spots on his back, appeared several months ago. Now he had a discoloration on the roof of his mouth and several more on his chest and legs. The lesion on his forehead appeared a few weeks ago and Sabir told me that when he saw it he completely panicked. He went to the pharmacy and spent an hour in the makeup section trying to choose a product that would cover it up but match his own dark skin coloring. The makeup department had astonished him with its vastness and variety. He hadn't smiled until that point but he gave a slight flicker of a smile as he told me how much it surprised him to realize that the whole world of makeup even existed. He knew his sisters wore makeup and he marveled that they navigated those aisles in the store with complete confidence. "I had no idea. I mean my sisters are each very beautiful and I know that they apply things to their eyes and their lips. I don't know how they could possibly choose from all of those little jars and pots."

His parents and sisters knew that Sabir had boyfriends but he worried that they'd reject him if they found out that he was sick with "that gay disease." Sabir remained close with his family although he harbored a lot of anger at his father, who'd been physically abusive when the children were young. While still possessed of a fierce temper, the father no longer hit anyone; he spent most of his days watching television or playing cards with his friends. He rarely spoke to his son. Sabir's sisters were older, and although they didn't criticize his lifestyle they did not include him in their social circles. "I just can't deal with this," he said of the mark on his forehead. "I want it to be gone. I wish I'd never been tested. Coming here was almost impossible for me."

Examining Sabir, I found several slightly raised dark purple patches, each about the size of a poker chip, on his back, with other lesions scattered on his chest and legs. In addition to the spot on the roof of his mouth he had thrush as well. Sabir couldn't tell me his T cell count but I guessed that it would be low.

Kaposi's sarcoma scared people. Patients died in much higher numbers from PCP, but it could be labeled "bronchitis" or "pneumonia" or some other euphemism to avoid saying "AIDS." A KS lesion might be passed off as a bruise for a few days but ultimately it was the hallmark of "gay cancer." The skinny guy covered with purple spots became the unwilling mascot of the dreaded epidemic. Before HIV, in previously described cases of KS the lesions typically appeared on the legs. Initially known only as an uncommon cancer occurring in elderly men from the Mediterranean basin, it was later recognized as an endemic form of childhood cancer in parts of Africa. Cases of PCP and KS were described in gay men who had unexplained immunosuppression in one of the first medical journal articles on HIV in 1981. The aggressive, disfiguring KS of the AIDS epidemic started as little painless spots, usually somewhere on the skin. As the number of cases of KS grew, it became apparent that the lesions could occur virtually anywhere on or in the body.

After I examined Sabir and ordered his blood tests, I made arrangements for him to see the radiation oncologist. Radiation would not treat the overall condition but could provide some cosmetic relief of individual lesions. First he needed a biopsy, as the oncologists would want to have a definitive diagnosis of Kaposi's sarcoma. As obvious as the diagnosis seemed, the oncologists needed pathologic proof before starting treatment. I called my colleague in the dermatology clinic to make sure that the biopsy would be done in the next few days and I made an appointment for Sabir to be seen across the street at the cancer hospital, where a colleague was working on new treatments for Kaposi's. Finally, I wrote Sabir prescriptions for medication to treat his thrush and started him on a daily dose of an antibiotic to prevent him from getting PCP.

We got up and I walked him back out to the waiting room. "The nurses will call you shortly to do the blood tests up here in our lab and the social worker will also meet with you today. Sabir, I want to see you again in two weeks."

He looked down and I worried that he would not come back. I shook his hand again then and told him, "You are doing the right thing now to be coming here. Please, I hope that you'll come back."

"OK," he said, looking briefly up at me.

I went back into my office and the secretary buzzed to tell me that Peaches had called and insisted that she speak to me. She would not say why she was calling, only that it was very important that I call back. The secretary gave me the number.

It had been many months since I'd seen her. She'd lost her food stamps but I was more afraid that she'd lose those young boys of hers; she couldn't leave the crack smoking behind her. The social worker had helped get her food stamps back. I wondered why she hadn't been coming to the clinic and what might be causing her to call now. The phone rang six or seven times before someone picked it up. I could hear a tremendous amount of noise in the background, obscuring a voice that said hello. It sounded like a gunfight taking place on the other end of the line, complete with blasts and shouts. "Hello?"

"Peaches?"

"Hello?"

"Peaches, it's Dr. Ball," I nearly shouted. Now I could hear screaming, live voices, laughter, as well as the recognizable blaring of a television.

"Hold on," I heard her say, and then "WILL YOU SHUT THE FUCK UP? MY FUCKING DOCTOR'S ON THE PHONE!" It didn't seem that she'd made any effort to cover the mouthpiece of the phone. I winced and held the earpiece away from my head. The screaming laughter subsided and the noise of the television diminished.

"Doctor Ball, I'm dyin'."

"Peaches, why do you say that? What's going on? Where've you been?" I didn't have her chart but my computer said that she hadn't been to the office in a year.

"I'm dyin', Dr. Ball, WILL YOU FUCKING SHUT UP?" The screaming had started again but quickly stopped.

"I haven't seen you in months, Peaches. Can you come in for an appointment?"

"I gotta come in. I gotta see you. TYRELL, WILL YOU GET THE FUCK OUT OF THERE? I'M GONNA FUCKIN' HURT YOU IF YOU FUCKIN' DON'T STOP FUCKIN' AROUND."

"Are you OK? Are the boys OK?" I don't think I'd ever heard anyone swear as much as Peaches. It certainly didn't sound like she was dying.

"Oh yeah, shit, they're driving me crazy. They're fine. It's me that's bad. I'm losing weight, I can't stop scratching everywhere, I don't even wanna smoke no more and you know that I gotta be dyin' if I don't wanna smoke." I could hear her give a little laugh over the sound of the gunfire on the TV.

"But where've you been? Have you seen a doctor at all? Do you still have the home attendant for the boys?"

"Hell yeah, that nurse still comes every week to bug the shit out of me. I ain't seen any other doctor. She told me to call you a month ago but I didn't want to. Shit, I didn't want to today either but I must be dyin' with all this scratching and the damn red blotches everywhere and GODDAMMIT TYRELL MY FUCKING DOCTOR'S ON THE PHONE WILL YOU SHUT THE FUCK UP OR DO I HAVE TO COME OVER THERE? Sorry, they just driving me crazy today."

"But why aren't they in school?" I was thinking, should I call the police? Is this routine for her? The TV racket and the yelling boys sounded like a Wild West shootout.

"Oh, the two big boys is in school but Tyrell had a earache this morning and Myron just had to keep him company. They fine, they be back in school tomorrow. Can I come tomorrow to see you?"

Tomorrow already looked jammed but she might not come if I made her wait. And with the way she was yelling I didn't want to say anything to irritate her further. "Sure," I said. "Come at one o'clock if you can. You might have to wait if it's very busy. But come in. It's been too long since you last came to see me."

"OK, I'll come. Thanks," and as the phone clattered down I heard the word "FUCK" once more. I hung up and looked around my office. It seemed very neat and quiet. Peaches's call felt like a desperate hand reaching for help out of thick pandemonium. Peaches, surrounded by noise and bodies but all alone and scared. She and Sabir lived in circumstances that might have nothing else in common, but both, like so many, were sadly isolated in their struggle with AIDS.

Someone knocked on my door and Jean, who had taken over Suzette's position as head nurse, stuck her head in. "John A. died."

"Oh." We looked at each other sadly. I could picture him so clearly with his blow-dry hairdo and those lovely hands waving around while he talked. John of the immaculate manicure. Taken by ambulance to a hospital close to his home about six weeks ago, once he was in the hospital his insurance did not allow him to transfer to us. A couple of times I spoke to the doctors there to give them John's history of PCP and collapsed lungs along with his medication list and recent lab results. I even talked to John himself from his hospital bed a couple of weeks ago when he'd improved and it looked as if he'd soon be going home. But then a big setback put him back in the ICU of the other hospital. Now this.

"Yeah," said Jean making a glum face. "I thought you'd want to know. His sister called Briana just now."

"Oh, that is sad news. Does she have the sister's number? I'd like to call her. Wasn't he such a sweet fellow?" I tried to think of the last time I'd seen John. I couldn't remember if it had been in the hospital or in my office. He had talked about going to hear some music in a church. It sounded beautiful and I'd briefly thought of trying to go and listen myself. But I couldn't recall any more details and I hadn't seen him again to ask about it. Now I would never know. Last year I tried to get him into a drug trial for one of the new medications, rumored to be a great breakthrough in treatment, but John had had too many episodes of PCP in his medical history and they didn't allow him to participate. I wondered, not for the first time, when or if we'd ever be able to treat this illness. Would John still be here if he'd gotten into the study, or were these new drugs going to disappoint us again? Would AIDS always be a death sentence?

After Jean left I sat there thinking about John while the surreal conversation with Peaches reverberated in my head. John's soft voice and fastidious mannerisms were like quiet pools compared to the rapids of Peaches's bellowing four-letter words and the chaos of noise in her house. I had to laugh; *shut the fuck up my fucking doctor's on the phone.* Yet where had she been? Her T cells were low a year ago, they couldn't be any better now. Why John and not Peaches? Allergic to Bactrim, which could protect him from PCP, John had been hospitalized several times with *Pneumocystis*. I didn't know why Peaches never got PCP; she didn't take her Bactrim even though she didn't have an allergy to it. Well, I'd find out more tomorrow. Hopefully she would show up. But I would never see John again. Another death to add to all the many losses. I wanted to get home to hug my little boy. I looked at my watch and got up from my desk to head to rounds.

Walking down the hall I thought again of Peaches's language. Later that evening I would call my mother in Florida to check on her and I'd probably tell her the story. I could just imagine my mother's voice on the phone saying, "Oh, Suze, really?" These days I spoke to my parents nearly every night. I looked forward to the calls, but the hollow thud in my stomach reminded me why I'd called them. My mother had been diagnosed with lung cancer less than a year ago when an abnormality was seen on an X-ray for a sore shoulder. A blur of tests and terrible apprehension and then the horrific diagnosis. For several months she did well, but things were accelerating now and her prognosis wasn't good. I visited them as much as I could, flying to Florida and back. I called often. She and my father would both get on the phone at once and let me know how things had gone that day; she was taking some mild chemotherapy that was geared to slowing down an inexorable process. They'd give me the weather report in Florida and relate the latest doctor's appointment or cancer clinic visit. Dad always told me of his fishing success, or lack thereof. Mostly we talked about Jules. My mother was happiest to hear some detail of her grandson's day, how he'd tried ice cream for the first time or how he'd still not gotten any teeth. I often told her about things that happened at CSS as well. For them, my work seemed completely foreign, a strange illness and entirely odd patients. My parents had no medical background whatsoever. They were intrigued, appreciative, and sympathetic and sometimes they were shocked or amused by the people I dealt with and the things that happened. I never named names, of course; I just described the personalities.

These days we talked more about work just because I talked to them so often. It provided an excellent distraction to have a colorful cast of characters to describe. What if I'd been a bond trader? Yeah, we put a bid on four thousand shares, yeah, that was so wild. No, I would tell them about my conversation with Peaches. My mother would be appalled by all the swearing but she'd want to know what was going to happen. Even without being a doctor, she would ask me thoughtful questions regarding how I was going to help

Peaches. I called my parents to comfort and support them but I found, not surprisingly, that I received some comfort and support in return.

Dan, one of my new colleagues, sat at the big round table chatting with a couple of the social workers when I got to rounds. Gerald was just starting to go through the list. I looked around the room and realized that there were more new faces than old ones. As people continued to come in and sit down, I took a seat next to Katie, one of the five or six new social workers who had come to work at CSS in the last two years. Since I'd started my job in 1992 approximately half the staff had changed. The patient load continually increased and the waiting list for patients wanting to get their HIV care at CSS grew longer. More and more people sat at the table for rounds. The clinic steadily evolved; we were like a city bus with new patients coming and others departing, new providers joining and others moving on. Dr. Jacobs, Stan, and I remained, and Gerald, Molly, Jean, and Sister Harriet as well. The biggest turnover took place among the social workers, although Warren's was the only position that had needed a replacement because of death. We had new nurses, new social workers, and a great nutritionist.

The biggest change for me was the departure of Maggie and the hiring of her replacement, followed not long after by our hiring a fourth doctor. When I started at CSS, Stan, Maggie, and I covered nearly all the patients; we knew one another's styles, strengths, and weaknesses. We covered one another and talked to one another's patients almost every night on call. A new doctor had so much to learn before he or she could really have a sense of knowing the patients and how all of us worked together. New faces and new personalities affected all of us, but a change in nurse or social worker didn't affect me as much as a new doctor.

Maggie's decision to leave came not long after her trip to Greece. She had had a difficult stretch with several patients dying in a short period of time and her heart seemed strained by her long-distance relationship. She'd gone back for a brief visit two months after they first met. When she announced that she wanted to stop working at CSS I felt relieved for her. Maggie sometimes gave too much and suffered for it, but her example was one of consuming dedication, a tough act to follow. While leaving seemed the right thing for her to do, I knew that her patients would miss the intense devotion with which she cared for them. All of us working at CSS recognized her selfless example.

Dan, hired to replace Maggie, came from Ohio, straight out of his residency, a former military officer dismissed under "Don't Ask, Don't Tell."

He assumed all of Maggie's patients and spent a few months adjusting to the schedule and the workload, and to the general embrace of working at CSS. Dr. Jacobs, Stan, and I took Dan out for cocktails one night to grill him on his sex life. Entirely in fun, it seemed a good way to warm him up to the closeness and collaboration of the CSS environment. We didn't know at the time why he'd left the military. Blushing fuchsia, he tried to avoid the questions, but Dr. Jacobs can be fairly persistent. One round of gin martinis led to the truth. Dr. Jacobs always referred to Dan as "Captain" after that evening. Dan's empathy and compassion stood out. His easygoing personality fit in with the team and, most important, the patients liked him very much.

Some months after Dan took over Maggie's patients we hired Brandon, whose new practice grew rapidly. Brandon also came right out of residency but in his pre-medicine life he'd been a trial lawyer. The multidisciplinary approach to patient care that formed the core of CSS didn't exactly resonate with Brandon, a fact that took us a while to grasp. He could be charming, warm, and friendly but unfortunately, with the social workers and the nurses, he could be arrogant, dismissive, and rude. In the nonhierarchical environment of CSS he rubbed a number of people the wrong way, something that hadn't ever really happened before. Brandon usually came late to the post-clinic conference and paid minimal attention. He didn't value the purpose of those rounds and sat reading his mail while others spoke. His attitude completely antagonized Gerald, who couldn't stand him and would have fired him happily. Brandon took good care of his patients, though, and as a peer he didn't bother Stan, Dan, or me in the same way he did the others. Our unit worked as a team and none of us approved of Brandon's treating the non-MDs dismissively. Dr. Jacobs didn't like Brandon's arrogance but did not intend to fire him.

Brandon did, however, wear white bucks with us on Fridays in the summer. When I was growing up my father wore white bucks to parties at the golf club we belonged to in upstate New York. Occasionally he'd have my sister and me paint them when they got too scuffed up. I had started wearing white bucks in college and still wore them at work occasionally in the summer months. One Friday at inpatient rounds, Dr. Jacobs and I were both wearing white bucks. Dr. Jacobs told Stan and Dan that they should get white bucks and we should all wear them on Fridays. Stan wore the same pair of shoes every day regardless of the season or the weather: he wore brown bucks with red soles. At Dr. Jacobs's suggestion Stan raised his eyebrows and said, "No fucking way." The next Friday, Dan showed up in white bucks and Dr. Jacobs had a box of size thirteen white bucks under his arm as a gift for

Stan. Stan put them on. The four of us stood there grinning at one another. We may have had no medicine to offer our patients, we may have lacked weapons or armor for the battles we waged, but at least we had our white bucks. Brandon thought we were nutty but after two or three weeks he arrived on a Friday wearing bucks. White ones.

Today as rounds got started my beeper went off. The number indicated a phone in the emergency room. This nearly always meant a patient needed admission to the hospital. I wondered which one it might be. I hoped it wasn't Cecil. With a pang I knew it wouldn't be John with PCP again. For some reason I thought of Hank. I pictured his tall lanky frame and the toilet paper stuffed in his ears and nose and wrapped around his penis. I hadn't seen him since the pharmacist called me to report the forged prescriptions. Where had he gone? I left rounds to answer the phone.

"Hi, Dr. Ball, your patient Sabitha L. is down here."

She had been at home for less than a month. The visiting nurses had called a few times to keep us up to date so I knew that her neurological function was deteriorating. I remembered the sad picture she and her boyfriend made as he wheeled her down the hall in her wheelchair. I also remembered the gorgeous young girl she'd been when I first met her just a year ago.

"She's been at home for the last several weeks," I told the ER resident on the phone. "What got them to bring her in?

"The boyfriend's with her. She can't speak very well but she's awake and alert. He says they just can't take care of her at home. Apparently she's not been eating much at all, she's too weak to get to the bathroom or to even tell them when she has to go. He almost looks worse than she does; he looks exhausted. She looks a little dehydrated but aside from the neuro stuff she seems stable."

"Poor thing," I said, thinking about the four young kids in her house. Sabitha, at fourteen, had been a child herself when her oldest, a girl now eleven, was born. Children having children.

"Is this HIV encephalopathy?" the resident asked.

"Yes, neuro thinks it's probably a combination of PML and HIV encephalopathy. Did you scan her?"

"No, the scanner's down right now, there are three people down here waiting for scans. I sent for her old chart. Her boyfriend told me about her history. He said her mother's completely alcoholic and unhelpful and he thinks Sabitha would be safer if she weren't at home. He seems like a pretty together guy."

"Yeah," I said. "He's been great considering how sick she's gotten. We talked to them about a nursing home before she went home last time." I felt glad her boyfriend remained in the picture. I remembered that in addition to being an alcoholic, the mother had a violent history. Sabitha once told me that her mother had been in jail in the past for assaulting someone with a knife.

"Dr. Ball, I read about some new medicine for AIDS patients. Is that something they could get?"

"Well, it's not available yet but the studies are looking very good. We're all hopeful."

"So there's not really anything to do for her?"

"No. We'll admit her. If she does need to go to a nursing home it'll be easier to get her in if she's here in the hospital. I'll be down to see her in a bit. Thanks."

I hung up the phone and put my head down on the desk. I had to get back to rounds but for a moment surge of sadness bubbled up in me like a shaken bottle of carbonated beverage. So did faces. I thought of Sabir, a new patient to me, obviously with advanced disease and a family situation that made him very isolated and alone. I thought about José, with his testosterone-infused muscles and dozens of tattoos, frantic if he had to spend more than five minutes in the waiting room with the other patients. He'd stand at the secretaries' credenza and ask them over and over when I would see him. Or another patient, Loretta, still drug-free, coming faithfully to her appointments, worried if her T cells dropped by 10 points, elated if they went up, pulling her life back together after crack. I thought about Peaches, frantic at home with her kids, screaming at them, screaming her fear and desperation. They all seemed alone. They all struggled in their different ways with having a disease for which they were often shunned, even by their own families. I had several patients who had never told anyone about their HIV diagnosis, not a friend, not a sibling, no one. For some, CSS offered the only respite from their extreme isolation.

I blocked my mind from thinking of my mother. I just couldn't let myself think of her while I was thinking of all of my patients. It would hit me later, after work. This sadness with my head on the desk came from today, from my patients, from AIDS and the fiery gash it caused across all these people's lives. The sadness for my mother came from a different place in my heart, a more primal one, wrapped in my childhood and my past. I would unwrap it and look at it later, as I did every day.

Meanwhile Sabitha lay on a stretcher downstairs in the ER, her scan showing a brain shriveled and pocked with white blotches. She couldn't walk, could barely speak, was going to be admitted and from here would go to a nursing home, where she would more than likely die. It stunned me still, this disease that could take a voluptuous, gorgeous young woman and in a year turn her into an old lady who needed diapers and someone to feed her. Was there really new medicine coming? Would it help? Could it possibly help someone like Sabitha? I lifted my head up from the desk, stood up, and went down the hall back to rounds.

"Doreen is doing fine, no problems today," I heard Brandon say as I sat down in one of the big leather chairs. Gerald didn't look up from writing on the interdisciplinary sheet but I saw him shake his head. Brandon rarely said anything other than so-and-so's doing well today, no problems. It infuriated Gerald.

Doreen's social worker, Kati, spoke next. "Doreen and I talked about her husband getting out of jail. He's been upstate for the last seven years. Apparently he doesn't know that Doreen has HIV and she doesn't know how to tell him."

"Is the husband infected?" asked Gerald.

"She says no. He would have been tested, of course, in prison, and she thinks he would have told her."

"So she didn't get it from him." Gerald looked over at Brandon, who was reading his mail. "Do you know how she got infected?"

Brandon looked up. "What?"

"How did Doreen get HIV? Do you know?"

"From her boyfriend. Her husband's in jail but he's coming home in a month or so. He doesn't know about the boyfriend." Brandon went back to reading his mail.

Gerald looked back at Katie, who nodded. "Well, that's basically what she told me, too, and now she's not sure what to do. She hasn't told him in all this time and now he's coming home." A couple of people around the table rolled their eyes.

"Is she afraid of him or anything?"

"No, no, he's not violent. But the boyfriend is not happy. He's living in Doreen's house now and says he isn't going to leave when the husband comes home." Now a few people muttered "oh great" or "uh-oh." Katie looked down at the papers in her lap. "She has a case manager on the outside who's hooked up with HASA and Morningstar and they are all aware of the situation. I suggested to Doreen that she at least let the husband know before he gets out of jail and shows up at their house. I'm not sure she'll follow that advice but it seemed the best option."

"OK," said Gerald. "Next we have Penelope P."

Stan leaned back in his chair and put his hands behind his head. "Penelope, as most of you know, is the former Peter P. and has now started her hormone injections and has started wearing a full wig and lots of makeup."

"And jewelry," someone down the table said.

"And lots of jewelry," said Stan, nodding. I knew exactly who he was talking about. A tall black man, Peter had been a patient at CSS from the start, a very flamboyant gay man who was a friend of Darren's, the guy with the Christmas tutu. Peter, recently transformed into Penelope, now clomped around in size thirteen pumps and sported heaps of gold bangles and rings and necklaces.

"Penelope's doing fine," Stan went on. "Apparently she has quite a reputation among her consorts. They call her Madame Medical Center."

Gerald was smiling as he wrote furiously on the sheet. "I hope she is modeling good behavior."

"Oh yes, she told me she is always very careful and lets no one near her if they aren't wearing a condom."

"What about you?" asked Gerald and the whole room laughed.

"Very funny." Stan chuckled. "She had some thrush today so I started her on Diflucan. And checked her labs."

"I saw Penelope today" came from Jeff, across the table. "I'm not sure but I think she was making a pass at me." Jeff's face became quite red as more laughter came from the group. "She kept petting my arm and calling me 'honey.'" I looked over at Stan who caught my eye. Jeff had recently been hired as a new social worker and Stan's glance agreed with me that neither of us was sure whether or not Jeff would actually be unhappy with Penelope's advances. "Her Medicaid is fine and she said she wants to work off the books at some bar downtown. I didn't get the details."

"No, better not to," said Gerald, looking up.

Rounds continued. The voices wove themselves around one another as the patients' names were called one by one. I talked about Sabir and the others I had seen in the clinic. It had been a long day. Afterwards I spoke to Katie, Peaches's social worker, to let her know that Peaches should be coming tomorrow. I went back to my office to finish my notes from the day. Before I went down to the emergency room to see Sabitha, I called John A.'s sister.

It bothered me that John had died in another hospital. I'd taken care of him through numerous complicated admissions; I knew him best. Once he was admitted to another hospital, however, I couldn't get him transferred unless our hospital offered something he needed that he couldn't get where he was, something like heart surgery or a brain biopsy. Sometimes, I admit, I was just as glad a patient could not be transferred. If I barely knew them or if I hadn't seen them in years, it didn't seem reasonable to transfer a patient simply because he knew my name and wanted to come to the medical center. This hadn't been the case with John, though. Another hospital could take care of John's PCP and collapsed lungs, but I felt unhappy not to be a part of his care. Occasionally patients got up and left where they were and came to our hospital still wearing their identification bracelet from the previous one. John was much too sick to do something like that and he lacked the extra thousand dollars to pay for a transfer on his own.

I dialed the number.

"Hello?"

"Hi, this is Dr. Ball. Is this Linda?"

"Yes?"

"Linda, I don't know if you remember me, we've spoken in the past but it was months ago. I was John's doctor at the medical center."

"Oh yes, of course, I remember. Dr. Ball, yes, of course."

"I'm just calling to tell you how sorry I am to hear that John is dead. And to thank you for letting us know. I really appreciate it. Everyone here appreciates it." I didn't like the euphemisms for death. Everyone says "passed away" or someone "passed" or "we lost them." It's not what happens. People die and then they are dead. They're gone, they're not lost. "Passed away" sounds unconvincing but "death" is not beating around the bush. "Death" is no more, not ever. I don't think it's gentle or kind to say "he's passed on," although I understand that some people need this as a way to avoid stating the obvious. The very young daughter of one of my friends once said, "When you're dead you're dead." And sadly enough, it's true.

"Oh, well, thank you, John always spoke so highly of you all."

"John was such a special guy. I'm very sorry."

"He was sorry that he couldn't get back to the medical center; he didn't like where he was. No one knew him there and it just felt different with the nurses and everything. He was all alone there."

"I'm sure. I'm sure that was hard on him, and on you, too. I just wanted to offer you and your family my condolences."

"Dr. Ball, he was the sweetest man I ever knew. He was beautiful."

I had a vivid picture in my mind of John of the immaculate manicure holding forth on some important tip on eyebrow tweezing. So earnest. I saw him clearly, lying propped up in his hospital bed, waving and floating his hands and talking in a gentle, quiet voice.

"We are going to miss him. Please convey our sympathies to the rest of your family. And please call if you need anything."

"Thank you."

And I hung up the phone realizing I'd probably never speak to her again, maybe never have an occasion to speak of John again.

# Chapter Thirteen

# 1996 Some Hope in the Despair

"Etta was admitted ten days ago with PCP. She spent five days in intensive care initially getting worse with treatment. She improved and went to the floor but earlier this week she developed fevers again and grew yeast in her blood. She's on IV fluconazole for that now as well. Overall she's better but her T cells are twelve and she's refused to take any medicine offered her as an outpatient. She's been too sick to protest here in the hospital but now that she's feeling better she's starting to refuse things again and I'm concerned that if she gets well enough to discharge she's not going to last long." I looked up as I ended my recitation.

"Nursing?"

"Etta's afebrile this morning and sat up in a chair last night." Judy looked down at her clipboard. As she continued her report I thought back on the time during my pregnancy when Etta insisted on going home from the emergency room to do her laundry despite her life-threatening anemia. Eventually she came in for a blood transfusion but even after that she wouldn't take iron to support her blood count. She'd give me one of those sneering looks of hers, as if saying, "What are you bothering me with this shit for?" then say she didn't need anything. She did take notice of her continued weight loss, however. For some overweight people the transition from a size eighteen to a size eight generates a fantasy of a magazine advertisement for magic weight reduction, but our patients don't mean to advertise HIV as a weight-loss formula. In Etta's social circle of hard drinkers and people in low-paying jobs, only the real losers used drugs, and HIV was something for the weird gay guys. Etta didn't do drugs and she thoroughly resented that people in her neighborhood assumed that her weight loss meant she had become a "crackhead." Of course HIV was in her community, yet there was so much stigma and secrecy around AIDS that she didn't worry as much about her real diagnosis being discovered.

But not even weight loss got her to take her medications. Etta persistently treated her HIV as an annoyance more than a concern. My efforts to get her to take her illness more seriously, to keep her appointments, to take the medications I prescribed for her always fell flat. Now it was early summer and her attitude was catching up with her in a bad way.

Etta lived in an apartment above her grandparents with her six-year-old son, Joey. About ten days ago the grandfather called upstairs and the little boy answered the phone saying Mommy was sick and couldn't get off the couch. The grandfather called CSS and an ambulance was sent to her house. I saw her in the emergency room, where she struggled to breathe despite the oxygen mask. She admitted that she'd never taken the Bactrim I'd prescribed for her, not even three times a week. Even with years of low T cells, until this admission she'd never had an opportunistic infection. Before now she'd never gotten anything but skinny and anemic. We could probably treat her PCP this time but what about the next time? The yeast in her blood shouted like a carnival barker that her immune system couldn't handle much of anything at all. Still, Etta made her own decisions. Now that she was improving she'd regained a good deal of her feistiness. When the nurses came to check her vital signs in the middle of the night she told them to get lost and complained to me about it in a disparaging tone when I saw her in the morning.

After inpatient rounds ended I went to see her. She was sitting in an armchair next to her bed wearing a pink bathrobe and fluffy pink slippers. Tubing ran down into her arm from the three intravenous bags hanging from the pole. On the lunch tray in front of her I saw she'd eaten some soup and part of a turkey sandwich. She stared at the television up on the wall opposite the bed. I glanced at it and saw one of those talk show hosts who gets people to cry or fight or both on the air. The camera panned to an obese woman who held the hand of a much younger, very skinny man. Both were crying.

The caption read "Son wants to marry his mother." Etta's mouth hung partly open as she watched the screen. When she saw me she gestured toward her lunch tray and in an aggrieved tone said, "I can't eat this. The food here really sucks." Then she looked back at the television.

I motioned for permission to sit down on her bed and she nodded. Picking up the TV remote, I asked if I could turn down the volume. Etta turned to me and then looked back at her food disgustedly. "I'm not kidding, this stuff is nasty. And I'm hungry for a change. My grandfather's bringing food later."

"Great. We always say that the patient is getting better when she starts complaining about the food here. It's a kind of test."

"Yeah, well, look at this soup." She picked up her spoon and dipped it into the glutinous orange liquid in the little plastic container. Appetizing it was not.

"Etta, you look great. So much better. And no fevers, right? How is your breathing?"

"It's fine. I'm fine. I'm ready to go home."

I almost laughed. A laugh of relief that she was better and a laugh at how crabby and tough she could be. "Listen, it's going to be a few more days. You're doing great, I'm really glad, but we've got to continue the IV for a little while more."

She made a *tsk*ing noise with her mouth and rolled her eyes. She looked back up at the television.

"Etta, once we stop the IV you're going to need to take pills. The treatment course for PCP is twenty-one days of antibiotics and so far you've had eleven days. The yeast in your blood can also, we feel, be treated with pills, but you're going to need to take them for a long time, maybe forever."

She turned toward me, a familiar, put-out look on her face. "Forever?"

"As long as your T cells are this low your body can't fight off the infection and so you'll need this medicine." She looked back at the television without saying anything. I went on. "There's some new HIV medicine also, and I want you to take it."

"*More* pills?" She looked as if I'd stabbed her.

"Yes, more pills. It's going to be a lot of pills. The new medicine is something we've been waiting for. It's called saquinavir." Later in the summer I was going to the International AIDS Conference in Vancouver. I looked forward to seeing the presentations and hearing the details of the studies on these new HIV medicines from the best AIDS researchers in the world.

She sneered. "I don't want to be a guinea pig."

"I know you don't. The testing has been done, the trials and everything. The government approved it and now you can get it in the pharmacy. You won't be a guinea pig."

"So how many pills are we talking about?" She looked up at the television again.

"A lot. Several pills three or four times a day." I knew this sounded utterly ridiculous for someone who would not even take one pill three times a week, but she wasn't going to get more chances if she didn't start to turn things around at this point. "We'll get you started while you're here so you'll be used to everything before you go home."

I watched her for a bit to see what she'd say. She continued to watch the TV without looking at me. I glanced up and saw a small man running across the studio stage with a cameraman following close behind. After a while Etta said, "I'm not going to stop eating from this, right? I'm finally eating decent again."

I thought for a moment. "You know, that's a good question. I can't tell you for sure, although I haven't heard anything about that being a problem. Everybody's different, though, and we're going to have to see how you get used to things. How your body adjusts." I took her question as an encouraging sign that she might really consider taking medications. "The steroids that you're on now for the PCP are helping you have an appetite but I'm hopeful that as you continue to get better you're going to want to eat more without them."

I watched her face. Then I said, "Etta, this has been a really serious illness and I'm not sure if things will work out as well for you if you have to go through it another time." She looked down at her lap. "I don't know for sure that these new pills are going to help you get better but I know that if you don't take them you definitely will not get better. Your system has really taken a beating, especially in these last few weeks." I couldn't be positive but it seemed she was listening. My pager started beeping. I shut it off and we sat there for a while, neither of us saying anything. Etta hadn't looked back up at the television.

"So—"

She interrupted me. "I'm going to take the pills." She looked at her food tray, not at me.

"OK. Great." I paused, thinking that it would be better not to say any more right now. Neither of us spoke for a while. I stood up.

"This food really sucks, though. I'm going home."

"OK. I know. Soon." I smiled a little as I said it and walked out of the room.

Upstairs Stewart sat in one of the chairs by the elevator and looked up as I got off. His thin, scraggly hair needed a wash and he wore an expression of calamity. "Oh, Dr. Ball, you're here. Did they tell you about my leg?"

"No, Stewart, they paged me. Wait just a moment and I'll come back out." I went through the waiting area and the door to the corridor to find Mary Rose in the hallway. She told me that Stewart had shown up saying his leg had been bothering him for a week. She'd paged me after looking at it. "It's pretty swollen and red. He doesn't have a fever, though."

I brought Stewart back to my office and looked at his leg. His right calf was warm, swollen, red, and tender. Stewart looked like he was going to cry.

"Is it another blood clot, Dr. Ball? It's not another blood clot, right? Why would I have another blood clot? The last time I had a fever and I don't have fever so it couldn't be another one but what is it?"

"It looks like you have a blood clot." I looked at his leg and shut my eyes so that he wouldn't see me roll them. Damn! Another blood clot in his leg. With a sense of dread I realized it meant another stint in the hospital, and this time he'd need blood thinners forever. I braced myself inwardly, anticipating the wave of his repetitive questions and my unheard answers.

HIV, as a chronic illness, could predispose people to an increased risk of blood clotting. We'd seen an occasional stroke in a young person or tiny blood clots in the lung that caused pulmonary hypertension. Stewart had had a blood clot in his right calf a year ago and been treated for three months with a blood thinner after a week in the hospital. His tremendous anxiety during that admission infected the floor nurses and the residents. Everyone found his constant questions hard to take. Although I joked about needing Valium to care for him, at the same time I felt somewhat defensive of my patient. He could be difficult but he wasn't a bad guy; he was worried.

Now I said to him, "Well, listen, let me get you an ultrasound so we can know one way or another if it's a clot. It does look like a clot, Stewart, you made the diagnosis on your own. This started a week ago?"

"Yeah, about a week ago."

"You didn't bang it or fall or anything?"

"No." Stewart sat in the chair in my office looking down at his leg with his khaki pants pulled up over his knee. He'd taken off his sock and sneaker and his damp yellow toes wiggled as we both looked at them. It seemed vaguely obscene and I looked up at his face instead.

"But no fever." I said it more as a statement than a question.

"No. I don't need to be admitted, do I? If we know what it is I can just take Coumadin and then I don't need to be in the hospital. Can this be fatal? I mean what are the complications? I know last time you told me I could get a clot traveling to my lungs. I don't feel short of breath but you know, my ears have been clogged for a few weeks, do you think that's part of it?"

"We need to have them do an ultrasound. Then we'll know if there's a blood clot and we'll go from there."

"But I haven't had any fever!" His eyebrows rose up ever higher on his forehead.

"I know. Maybe this isn't a clot but for right now let's proceed as if it is. OK? We'll get an ultrasound. Let me make a few calls and then we'll see what we need to do. I think you should be in the hospital, though, with this."

"In the hospital?"

"Yes."

"Now?"

"Yes, now, Stewart. If it isn't a blood clot there's at least a skin infection going on which will need antibiotics. I think you'll probably need both heparin and antibiotics so let's assume that you need to be admitted. I'll set up the ultrasound and from there you'll go to the emergency room."

I almost jumped up from my desk, feeling that I could not bear to go through another round of the same questions. I cajoled him to get his sock and shoe back on and walked with him down to the lab to get his blood drawn before going for the ultrasound. Back in my office I made the arrangements for his admission. All the while I lamented the fact that now Stewart would need to be on blood thinners every day forever. We'd have to watch his medication levels, which meant he'd need to come to the lab on a regular basis. It was like anticipating indefinite weekly visits for orthodontia adjustment. I could imagine what the nurses were going to say.

Back downstairs on the inpatient floor I went to see Roman, a patient whom I'd met six months ago, sent from the office of a doctor friend of mine when Roman's insurance wouldn't cover his visits. Roman had one of the worst cases of Kaposi's I'd ever seen, chiefly because of how grossly the purple swelling deformed his eyes. Whereas Sabir's KS was sprinkled over all parts of his body, so far the lesions had barely touched his face. The confluent, violacious lesions that covered Roman's back didn't avoid his face. His eyelids and cheeks puffed with the puckered reddish-violet masses. He had no pain from these lesions but the disfigurement made life very difficult. He wore sunglasses everywhere but still people stared at him on the street. He told me that he felt as if he constantly carried a big blinking sign over his head that announced, "Watch Out, This Man Has AIDS!" Roman worked as the driver and handyman for a wealthy woman who well understood his story. It was her physician who had sent Roman to me. Her work in theater advertising involved dealing with lots of gay men and so HIV did not shock or repulse her; she'd seen plenty of it. She came to Roman's first appointment with him and continued to employ him despite his disfigurement.

Several weeks ago Roman developed shortness of breath and a cough, and I admitted him this week assuming that he had PCP. He refused to have the pulmonary doctors look down into his lungs to investigate the fluffy white patches revealed by his chest X-ray. Roman insisted that he never missed his Bactrim dose. It would be very unusual for him to have PCP if this were the case. I pressed him to have the bronchoscopy so we could know for sure. For a week I treated him with powerful medication against PCP, using something other than Bactrim. He didn't improve but his laboratory results and his symptoms seemed less like classic PCP. Our diagnosis shifted to the next likely illness, Kaposi's of the lung. I was worried.

I walked into the bright room with its view of the Empire State Building.

Roman was sitting up in bed wearing striped pajamas and horn-rimmed glasses, reading the *New York Times*, his white sheets and cotton blanket all neatly tucked in around him. He put his paper down.

"Dr. Ball," he said, with his lilting Brazilian Portuguese accent.

"How are you feeling?"

"I'm feeling OK." He smiled a bit, his eyes disappearing behind the purple swellings that crowded one another all over his face.

"Cough? Fever? Anything new?" I took my stethoscope out of my pocket.

"I'm coughing when I lie flat at night. I find that I'm sitting up more to be comfortable." He leaned forward and helped me lift up the back of his pajama top. He took some deep breaths in and out while I listened. Then he sat back against his pillows and breathed quietly while I listened to his heart. He knew this ritual well after a week. I draped my stethoscope around my neck and sat on the end of his bed.

"Well, you sound about the same to me. There are areas that don't move air so well. The X-rays haven't changed really at all in this week. Are you still sure you won't let anyone look down there?"

"You've said there's no treatment, only some chemotherapy that doesn't work."

"For KS you mean."

"Isn't that what you think it is?"

"Yes." I shifted as I sat there. "It's just that I don't *know* that that's what it is. I *think* it is. I think all other possibilities are pretty remote, given how much KS you have on your skin. But it's just white patches on the X-ray; it's not actual tissue to stain and really look at. Without that I can't say absolutely it's KS."

"Dr. Ball, you said you wanted to give me some new medicine for HIV."

He was changing the subject but I didn't mind. We'd been over the bronchoscopy issue more than a few times and he wouldn't budge. "Yes, I think we should get you started on the new medicine. Maybe if we get your T cells up a little they'll help fight against the KS. It's definitely worth a try." I'd hear the specifics in a few weeks at the Vancouver conference, but with FDA approval I didn't have to wait to start my patients on the new medicines. I just hoped that they'd work as well as the initial reports were claiming.

"OK. I'd like to get out of this hospital."

Roman seemed remarkably fine despite his alarming appearance and his nasty chest film. Short of breath if he moved around a lot; just sitting there in bed he had no complaints. Sometimes I wondered how, with their T cells in the single digits, some patients looked fit and healthy whereas others looked like skinny wrecks. I didn't kid myself about Roman's appearance. Patients with KS of the lungs did not survive for long.

"Roman, I need to ask you, with this whatever-it-is in your lungs, your breathing is already affected and there may come a time when you are unable to breathe on your own. I don't think that is going to happen today, but if you can't breathe on your own do you want to be placed on a breathing machine?"

He gave me a perplexed look. It appeared that this thought had not occurred to him before and I felt disappointed in myself that I had not brought it up until now. "This is something I should have spoken with you about sooner," I said.

He shook his head. "No it's not that, it's that Olaf died after being on a machine for four weeks. It was awful."

"I'm sorry, I didn't know. That was three years ago, right?"

He nodded. Neither of us said anything. I waited as Roman looked down and smoothed the blanket. After a bit I said, "If we aren't treating this thing in your lungs, I'm not sure that putting you on a breathing machine would serve a purpose. It could keep you alive but not indefinitely."

"What would happen instead?" He looked up at me and squinted through the purple swellings of his eyelids.

"We would keep you comfortable. We'd give you small doses of morphine so that you would not feel pain or feel anxious."

"And I would die?" He looked out the window past me and I watched his face, wondering what else there could possibly be to say.

Finally I said, "Roman, we just don't have a cure for this. Not yet. I will say, though, that the people taking the new medicine you're starting are doing super-well. This is not a done deal."

"I know I don't want to be on a breathing machine. Definitely not."

"OK, that's important for us both to know, and as I say, I don't think you are anywhere near being at that point right now. I've ordered the medication for you. It's a lot of pills but let's see if they can help."

"OK."

Months passed. I went to Vancouver and came back, as we all did, with an unfamiliar sense of optimism. This optimism contrasted sharply with how we usually felt after international AIDS conferences, when we came home decidedly glum as the numbers of cases always rose, the poor and needy suffered increasingly, and none of the treatments in development ever worked. This time the data on the new medications, the protease inhibitors, confirmed and augmented what our own clinical experiences were starting to show—that patients on these medications could do well. Finally, finally, a significant positive advance in the treatment of HIV. People were almost giddy with excitement.

September came. Etta stayed out of the hospital and Roman called for medication refills from his job in the Hamptons with the rich lady. At home Jules explored the sandbox in the park and loved being read to in the evening. We read the usual classics: Good Night Moon, A Fly Went By, Harold and the Purple Crayon. At less than two years old he didn't talk much yet and he tended to be shy with strangers. Our gray cat, Kitty, watched over him. My mother's cancer spread to her spinal cord and radiation therapy only proved exhausting for her. I was spending increasing amounts of time in Florida. By the early fall she could no longer get out of bed. I went back down to see her.

"Mom, give a cough."

She coughed a puny little cough. I didn't expect anything thunderous.

"That's good, cough a few more times." I couldn't see her face. She lay with her back to me and I stood at the side of the bed wearing surgical gloves, with one hand holding her hip and two fingers of the other hand exploring her rectum in order to help her move her bowels, something she hadn't done in a week or more. She hadn't asked me to do it. But she couldn't move or feel anything below her waist. The visiting nurses wouldn't do this, or maybe they weren't allowed to; I'm not sure.

"Poor Suze." Mom gave a low laugh as she said it. Her voice was muffled by the pillows around her head.

"What? Why poor Suze?"

"You have to change Jules's diapers and now this."

"Oh. Well, this isn't so bad, really." I almost had it. "Am I hurting you?"

"No."

"Can you feel it?"

"No."

"It's not the first time I've had to do this," I said. "I guess life isn't complete until you have manually disimpacted your own mother." I could hear the tone of my voice. I sounded relaxed. I tried to ignore the part of me that felt like hanging my head and crying. My son was not yet two and of course I changed his diapers. Yet I thought of my mother as discreet and elegant, not someone who needed this sort of help. Ever gracious and reserved, she calmly answered when I asked her about her bowels. She took such pride in my having chosen medicine for a career and if I, as her doctor daughter, recommended something she did not complain or object. We both understood that cancer was winning this battle.

"Lucky you." I heard her voice from the pillows.

"Lucky me."

"Who's lucky?" Margo came into the room and stopped. "What's going on?"

"I'm helping Mom poop. Mom, give a couple more coughs."

Each cough resulted in her muscles bearing down and after a few more I had delivered a soft little mass. Margo looked at me with raised eyebrows. "Eew." My sister worked in the accounting office at the exclusive Florida resort three miles up the road from my parents' house. She came over to the side of the bed where I stood. She looked and gave a little giggle. "It looks like a Tootsie Roll."

Mom's muffled voice answered, "Delightful. Don't eat it."

"Mom!"

This activity had produced the desired result so Margo and I cleaned her up and helped her roll onto her back. We lifted her to sit up against her pillows.

I sat down on the little chintz chair next to her bed and Margo stood at the end of the bed, watching Mom. Absentmindedly her hand rubbed her belly. A boy. She and Ray were having a boy. She had the name picked out and the room decorated. She had her baby car seat, a crib, and a high chair. She talked about onesies and birthing classes. Months ago my mother helped Margo with the maternity shopping and the planning for the new baby's room. Jules lived far away in New York and came for visits; she'd only once met the newborn son of my oldest brother, Fred, who lived in Virginia. This baby would be right here and it was hard to tell who was more excited, my mother or my sister. But as her cancer progressed, Mom's attention shifted. She didn't have pain and certainly she knew all of us, but the radiation and the brain lesions took their toll and part of her was leaving even now. It seemed she couldn't bring her thoughts to focus anymore, and none of us could talk of her missing the birth of a grandchild.

"Muggs, I'll sit here for a bit." Dad gave my sister her nickname years ago. "Dad's out fishing. Are you feeling OK? Do you want to stay for dinner?"

"No, I'm good. Ray is at home. We're going to a baseball game later. By the way, I can't poop either."

"Don't look at me."

Mom lay there with her eyes open, a few wispy hairs on her otherwise bald head, her misshapen jaw a reminder of another surgery six years before the cancer. What was she thinking now?

"Mom, Margo can't poop either."

"I heard."

"Want some more ginger ale?" I held out the can to her and put the straw to her lips. She took a couple of sips from the straw.

Margo came around and kissed Mom on the cheek. "Bye. I'll call you later."

"Bye, honey."

"Mom, try and eat something, OK?"

"I will."

"Sure." Margo rolled her eyes at me.

Mom wouldn't eat and we both knew it. I pushed her to drink but she refused to eat and I couldn't make her. It drove my father practically insane that she wouldn't eat. He'd get mad at her and start yelling, which didn't help and certainly didn't make her hungry. I found myself yelling at everyone else: at Dad, my brothers, my partner, at Margo. My yelling bounced off my aching heart and clanged around in my hollow chest. A dull, loud clanging. I saw myself waving my arms and shouting, hurling, desperate, desolate, no sound but the din in my ears. Standing on a cliff. Aren't we always standing on a cliff? She was leaving us. She didn't want to go, but some weeks ago, I don't know when, she'd found herself on a raft in a steady, ebbing current, swirling slowly, gently even, being borne away from us. She didn't wave. And so we sat with her. Day after day. In these last weeks I'd been in Florida a lot, just to sit with her. Dad couldn't bear it. He ran errands or dashed out to go fishing. He rummaged around in the garage and appeared in the bedroom doorway, his skimpy gray hair standing up on his head. "Everything OK?" he'd ask, and then he'd go out again.

Margo worked at her job and stopped by nearly every morning and every afternoon on her way home. My brother Jim and I tried to alternate our visits, coming down from New York to be with her. Fred could not come as often. I missed a lot of work. Sometimes I brought Jules with me for a few days. He found her bald head very curious and he patted it with his soft little hand. Although he knew very few words, he'd say "Granny" in a precious small voice. When he patted her head she looked at him with heart-aching pale blue eyes. She smiled with her misshapen face and her hands reached out to touch him. "Hello, Julot," she said.

I liked sitting with my mother. We sat together for many hours, often silently. Sometimes I read to her. Once, when sitting by her and holding her hand, I said, "Mom, you have been a good mother." She let go of my hand and reached up to put her arm around me and said, "Oh, honey, there's so much I want to say but I can't say it." And so I imagined that even though she tended to be so quiet she had many thoughts whirring through her head.

After Margo left I sat by the bed. I liked the comfortable little chintz chair next to her bed and I put up my feet on the matching ottoman to sit next to her. The TV on the dresser blinked without sound. We both watched the flickering screen. Sometimes I talked to her about the news. She listened to me and made an occasional comment. But she drifted away. She wasn't coming back. None of it mattered very much at all to her.

"Mom, you know I was in Vancouver this summer."

"Mmmm."

"I was there for a conference. The International AIDS Conference. Remember I went to Japan a couple of years ago?"

She seemed to be listening. I kept going.

"So it was very interesting this year. A bunch of us from work went. I had a presentation and work paid for us to go. There is some new medicine now for AIDS. It seems like it works very well. The patients in the studies who took the medicine stayed healthy and didn't get sick."

She licked her lips. I reached over with the can of ginger ale and she took a sip from the straw.

"I have a couple of patients on the new medicine. I have a patient named Etta. She's taking all these new pills. She's been hard to take care of because she has a mind of her own and doesn't do what I ask her to do."

Mom reached up to her lip and wiped at it with her finger.

"She has been super-sick. I really thought she was going to die this summer. I think of her because she has a little boy who is just a little older than Jules."

"Jules?"

"Yes."

"Oh, that's too bad." I wondered if she knew what I was talking about or if she was just responding to my voice saying the name of her grandson. I almost laughed. Should I just keep talking? Could she even say what she was thinking about? Was she suffering? Was she aware? All these questions went across my brain like a ticker tape. I had no answers. I looked down at the can of ginger ale in my hands and kept going with my story.

"It's sort of amazing, really. She's been on this medicine and she's doing better. I really thought that she was going to die. I always think of Jules when I see her and I worry about that little boy. So now I feel a little better because Etta is doing so much better. It's really been remarkable. Anyway, in Vancouver we heard about the studies on these new drugs and so we're all hopeful that there's something for our patients finally. Maybe everyone won't die now." When Etta had finally been discharged after a slow recovery from PCP, I had not been optimistic. She'd complained about all the pills she had to take in the hospital and I thought she'd stop them all once she got out. A month later, just before I left for Florida, she had an appointment with me. She complained about everything, but how delightful to see her ten pounds heavier, wearing glossy pink lipstick and her blue eye shadow once again. There could be no doubt that my patient was getting better.

Mom didn't say a word. She kept looking at the silent television.

"Vancouver is very beautiful. It's right on the water."

"Nice." Maybe that was all she heard. She loved the water. She loved their house in Florida, looking out over the water. Once when we were walking on the beach together, a few years ago, after they'd bought the house and moved away from the freezing, endless upstate New York winters, she said she felt so lucky to be able to be in that spot and to see the water every day.

I sat next to my mother and watched her face. Can I hold her here, I wondered, can I remember this moment and all its awful greatness? She is here next to me and I am holding her hand. She knows I'm here and my love surrounds her; I know she knows it does. Then I thought of Etta and realized that if not for the protease inhibitors Etta would most certainly be dead by now. Instead she was putting on makeup and complaining about her pills. Taking them, but complaining. No pill was out there for Mom.

I thought about my trip to Vancouver last July. I had rented a bike one day after the conference sessions and rode along the water on the bike path that circles Stanley Park. The park is full of the tall, dark pines of the Northwest. Moss and green ferns cover the forest floor and fallen trees. The bike path goes right under the Lions Gate Bridge. Huge ships coming into the harbor go through that narrow stretch with the bridge high overhead. They seem almost close enough to touch. As I rode along I saw a sailor standing far up above me, puffing on a cigarette, looking down at me from the rail of his enormous red ship as it passed under the bridge, heading out through the Lions Gate. I wondered where they were off to: somewhere to the west, to Asia maybe, or Australia. Maybe they were headed to Bora Bora or Tahiti. Around the northern end of Stanley Park the water opens out and there is no land on the horizon. I got off my bike and sat on the rocks looking far across at the blinding afternoon sun sparkling on the water. The big ship I'd seen with the smoking sailor headed out there, out to sea. The Pacific Ocean seemed vast and unknowable. I sat with my rented bike for a long time and watched the big red ship move slowly, steadily off, getting smaller and smaller. The light glinted and the water sparkled dark and brilliant.

Earlier that day I had called my parents at the Florida house. My mother's CT scan results were in. She'd already had radiation therapy to her brain in the spring. She couldn't get any more. After four weeks of radiation therapy to her spine she was done with that as well. It had thoroughly exhausted her. My father told me the results of the CT. His voice was quiet and sad. I hung up the phone in the hotel room in Vancouver. She still had evidence of cancer in her brain. I went outside and walked down to the harbor and rented the bike to go riding in Stanley Park.

Two months later I was in Florida with Jules, sitting by my mother's bed in the afternoons, watching the silent television while he napped. The summer tourists had gone back inland and the island enjoyed the golden days of early fall. I took Jules to the beach early every morning on my mother's bicycle to look for shells and watch the gulls. One morning the water fairly glowed in the first rays of the sun. We stood at the edge of the Gulf of Mexico. I held

Jules in my arms and he held his little orange rubber lion in his hand. The sun glanced up over the Australian pines behind us. We looked out at the bright green-gray water, watching for the fin of a dolphin. We'd seen one yesterday morning. Jules looked intently, his white-blond feathery hair lifting off his brow. The water gently curled in waves at my ankles, the smooth sand wearing away beneath my feet. Our shadows stretched out into the water in the first morning sunlight. A lone silhouette in the distance bent to pick up a shell. I put Jules down and he squatted on his little legs and poked at the sand, holding his lion carefully in his fist. We walked north along the edge where the sand has a ridge of tiny shells and gifts from the night tide. We found a whelk, bright orange, smaller than a peanut. We found a baby crab skeleton. We stood for a while watching the pelicans soaring and plunging into the gulf. Jules smiled and pointed. After a while more we went back to the house. Jules rode in his seat behind me as I pedaled.

# Chapter Fourteen

# 1996 Hit Early, Hit Hard

"Hit early, hit hard" became the mantra for HIV care after the presentations at the AIDS conference in Vancouver in 1996. What a strange, almost euphoric feeling, to think that now we finally had effective medication to treat our patients. Those of us who had started prescribing these medications had seen definite evidence of improved health in our patients and the presentations in Vancouver validated our experiences. The new family of drugs, protease inhibitors, when used in combination with other HIV medications already on the market, eradicated the virus from the blood. This in turn led to a rise in the T cell count and improved immune function. The word "cure" could be heard in various places regarding what these new regimens could mean for patients with AIDS. A cure for AIDS: what an amazing idea. We assumed that everyone should be taking these medications.

Before 1996 we could never measure the level or actual number of viral particles in the bloodstream, or whether our medications made that number go down. Previously, only T cell levels could tell us about the progression of disease; they were the surrogate marker for the effectiveness of medications like AZT. T cells are lymphocytes, one of several forms of white blood cells that participate in a properly functioning immune system. We use the terms T cells and CD4 cells interchangeably, but in fact CD4 cells are just one kind of T cell and they are the preferred target for HIV. HIV enters these cells and uses the host cell's DNA to replicate, killing the cell in the process. We knew that higher T cell counts meant a patient was not in imminent danger of opportunistic infections such as PCP or CMV retinitis. The protease inhibitors, our new weapon against HIV, came to market at a time when the technology had evolved and enabled us to measure exactly how much virus could be found in the blood. We could see direct effects of the medication, not just indirect effects. The amount of virus, what we called the "viral load," decreased to levels below the limit of detection when patients took the new protease inhibitor regimens. No virus detected. T cells going up. Hurrah!

Roman's face told an abridged version of the story. He smiled at my disbelieving look when he finally made it back from the Hamptons in October. For the first time I could see that his eyes were light brown. In the four months since he started taking his "cocktail" of new medications, the disfiguring purple swellings over his eyelids had faded. His eyelids remained slightly puffy and pink but it was as if the lesions had reversed course, like a flower blooming backwards. Roman had put on some weight, which lent an increased look of health to his handsome face. He brushed his fair hair back from his forehead and as he talked his breathing came easily; he never coughed. The pulmonary lesions on his chest X-ray had nearly disappeared as well. Roman told me that at first he'd found it very difficult to take the medication. He'd felt sick and the requirement to take the pills every eight hours on an empty stomach thoroughly disrupted his eating schedule. Gradually, he said, he adjusted. "I knew that I didn't have a choice." I asked him if he'd missed any doses. Not once, he said, never once.

Though remarkable, Roman's case was not unique. In these last months we'd seen several patients whose KS lesions had markedly faded since they started taking combination therapy that included protease inhibitors. Other patients with symptoms or conditions of advanced HIV improved on the medication as well. Those with profound wasting began to gain weight, those with unexplained rashes saw their skin clear up, and several patients reported their unremitting diarrhea had stopped within weeks of starting on a regimen with protease inhibitors. As I looked back at fifteen years of death and no effective treatments to offer, the changes at first seemed like illusions, as if conjured by magic. I almost felt that at any moment the "real" disease would rear up and devour my patients. But slowly I began to believe.

The blood tests supported this symptomatic improvement, revealing significant increases in T cell counts. Patients taking the "cocktail," as we began calling the combination of medications, took lots of pills, with lots of side effects, but showed slow, steady improvement in their immune systems. Most patients with low T cells also had hundreds of thousands of copies of virus per milliliter of blood. Some viral loads were in the millions. With the new technology we began to routinely measure viral load levels. We used the viral load assay to measure the amount of virus at the initiation of therapy. Once patients were on the medication for a few weeks these levels dropped so low the assay couldn't find any virus at all. Patients achieved undetectable viral loads. It was stunning.

And yet that time for me was and always will be marked by the sadness of my mother dying. My time involved lots of late nights and early mornings on airplanes back and forth from Florida, waking up in tears to hug Jules and Shari, rushing off to my office hours at CSS, and flying down to Florida to sit and hold my mother's hand. The blur of competing hope and despair, excitement and sadness, work life and family life kept me dizzy and tired. Dr. Jacobs never questioned my absences, and my colleagues covered for me time and again without the slightest hesitation. Stan's support came from the heart, I knew. His mother's cancer had been in remission longer than anyone had expected, with no signs of coming back. My mother's relentless course offered no respite. She died just before Thanksgiving. Shari and my brothers arrived the next day and shy Jules ran into my mother's room calling her name. "Granny," he said, stopping in the doorway, holding the little orange lion. "Granny?"

Back in New York, in December, at clinic rounds one afternoon Zoe Prin told us that one of her patients, a large African American woman, had stood up in the middle of their session and with grand gestures sung a loud a cappella verse of "O Come, All Ye Faithful." The exuberance and hopefulness of "joyful and triumphant" resonated throughout the days at CSS. We had clearly turned a corner in our ability to treat HIV. Success and recovery became very real possibilities, and the deep gloom of AIDS lifted with the stories of increasing T cells, returning appetites, and fewer cases of PCP.

Sabir came back to my office that month looking worse than ever. The single lesion that had marked his forehead when I first met him now spread down the side of his face. It looked like someone had glued dark, dense purple oatmeal to his head. The lesions on his back had become confluent masses that nearly obscured his normal skin. He had never gone back to the radiation oncologist to have the lesions treated, nor had he filled any of the prescriptions I gave him. He rarely missed an appointment with me, though, and I saw him almost monthly; at each visit he seemed worse. I struggled with my own sense of disappointment and even irritation when I offered treatment options, medications, pep talks, and encouragement and he refused all of it. I wondered if depression clouded his judgment and I asked one of our psychiatrists, Dr. Paul Ferand, to see him. He, too, offered a number of medications to try to lift the dark cloud of suffering but Sabir wouldn't take anything.

"I don't think he's clinically depressed," Paul told me one afternoon in the hall after he'd seen Sabir for the third time. "He's discouraged, which of course is understandable, but he's eating and sleeping and he's not suicidal or anything like that."

"So why does he refuse everything?" I asked him.

"Well, I'm not entirely sure," he said shaking his head and adjusting his wire-rimmed glasses. "He's help-rejecting, for sure, but not in that borderline way that some patients have. He's hopeless. I think that's more to the point. He has no hope."

"But I've tried hard to talk to him about the protease inhibitors. I told him about Roman, what a great recovery he's making. Sabir seems unwilling or somehow unable to make the connection that he could be that guy too if he'd take some medications."

"That's it, a bit, I think. His whole life he's separated himself from who he is. His father was this overbearing, really brutal guy and Sabir had to be someone else in order to get along in his house. He loves his father, but in order to live in his father's world he had to dissociate himself from his own world."

"You mean from being gay."

"Yeah," he said, nodding. "And so I think this is just a pattern for him and he's unable to connect to his illness."

"But all he has to do is look in the mirror." I could understand being distant from oneself, but oblivious?

"No, it's not that. He's aware that he's sick but at the same time he's not really experiencing it. It's almost like it's separate from him. Treating it would make him own it and that's more than he can take." He shook his head again, smiling sadly. "He needs a good psychiatrist."

Paul had years of experience taking care of people with troubled childhoods. He'd been working with our patients for more than two years. I sought his input and respected his opinions. Hearing this perspective on Sabir, I smiled and nodded. "It's hard for me that he's so adamant. Not adamant, that's not the right word. He's hopeless, as you say. All these other patients getting on meds and turning things around and he won't even try. What you're saying makes sense and I have to remember that it's not about me."

"Oh, no. Not at all. It's not about you."

Paul's words reminded me that Sabir's refusals were not personal. Sabir had a complicated way of dealing with the world and I appreciated hearing the psychiatric point of view.

Still, as Sabir sat down across from me, I had to fight back my own feeling that his refusal to take medicines or go to the radiation oncologist was wrong-headed, like wearing flip-flops in a snowstorm. Certainly he didn't act like he was fighting this thing; indeed he looked pretty wretched as he sat there with a scarf wrapped around most of his lower face and a hat with sheepskin ear-flaps pulled low over his eyes. His clothing looked too big. I could see a bit of purple on the small visible part of his face. The purple of defiance. Not Sabir's defiance, unfortunately.

"How are things going?" I asked him after he sat down.

"About the same." He looked at me from under the brim of his hat and his dark eyes gave away very little. He didn't hold my gaze and looked back down at his lap.

"Any fevers? Coughing? Headaches? Diarrhea?"

He shook his head at each question. "No, just these things getting bigger. The one in my mouth sometimes feels weird."

I had him sit up on the examining table and looked in his mouth and listened to his heart and lungs. I could see very little healthy skin on his back, covered as it was almost entirely by Kaposi's.

"Can I set you up to see the radiation people?" He shook his head even as the words came out of my mouth. "Medications?" Again the wordless no. I'd been over the options with him at each visit in the last four months. My lengthy explanations never changed his mind. Today I wouldn't start the whole spiel again. "How are things at home?"

He shrugged and got down from the table, wrapping the loose scarf around his face once again. "I moved back home."

He said it nonchalantly but he'd talked to the social worker and Dr. Ferand about this possibility. Far more than giving up a living space, giving up his apartment meant relinquishing his independence. I looked at him questioningly.

"It's fine. It's better. My apartment was too expensive." He busied himself with tucking in his shirt and didn't look at me. I stood there watching him and suddenly I had the urge to put my arms around him. He seemed so stuck in this dismal situation. What if he felt loved? What if someone reached out across all that imaginary barbed wire that he had woven around himself year after year? His eyes lifted again and met mine. "I'm at home with my family," he said, almost as if he knew what I was thinking and had come to the same conclusion. I felt a resigned smile come over my face.

My phone rang and I answered it.

"DOCTOR BALL, I'M DYIN'," came a very loud voice that I hadn't heard in a while but which I remembered well. How did she come to have the number of my private line?

"Peaches."

"I'M DYIN' AN' YOU GOTTA SEE ME."

"Peaches, listen, I'm with another patient right now. Can I call you back in a little while?"

"I'm in the waiting room, Dr. Ball. Just come and get me."

I hung up the phone and put my head back and closed my eyes. She was calling me from twenty feet away.

I looked over at Sabir who had heard every word. His eyes gave a little twinkle of complicity. I smiled and shook my head. "Sorry. That's a patient of mine."

"Is she really dying?"

"I hope not, but she doesn't keep her appointments very well so I'm glad she's here. Sorry for the interruption, though."

Sabir shrugged his shoulders and started putting on his coat, carefully adjusting the scarf to cover his face. Then he pulled it down from his mouth and said, "My mother wants to meet you. Is it OK if I bring her here?"

"Of course," I said, nodding at him and moving toward the door. "That would be fine. Is there anything that you don't want her to know?"

"No, she knows." He reached out and shook my hand. I usually shook patients' hands when I met them for the first time but not always after that. Sabir and I shook hands after every visit. I liked it. I wished Sabir would allow me to help him. With all his refusals I wondered why he kept coming to CSS, but we must have offered him something, as he rarely missed an appointment. Perhaps the general support of the team reassured him. No one freaked out looking at him. No one turned him away because he didn't do what we asked. I looked forward to meeting his mother.

Out in the hall Jean told me that Peaches was yelling at various people in the waiting area. "She's stuffing her face out there, eating two bagels at once, making a real mess and wiping her nose on her sleeve. Where's she been? She looks bad."

"Listen, I have two or three more people to see before I can see her. Is Briana around?"

Just then Briana, one of the social workers, came out of her office. "Is it about Peaches?"

"How'd you guess?" I asked as Jean shook her head with a little laugh and went back down the hall.

"I wanted to check with you first before I bring her back to my office," Briana said.

"I need to see a couple of people but it sounds like she's raising a ruckus out there so maybe if you aren't busy, yes, you could see her first. She called me at my desk from the waiting room to say she was dying!" Briana and I both started laughing. "The last time she did this she came the next day but then dropped out of sight again."

"I can see her now."

"That's great, thanks."

I went to the door of the waiting room and called Olive's name.

Peaches looked up from where she sat in an armchair on the far wall and yelled, "DR. BALL!" She had a mouthful of food and held a half-eaten bagel in one hand. Her hair, never tidy, stood up in bunches all over her head and from across the room I could see that she'd lost weight and her skin looked very blotchy. I let the waiting room door shut behind me and went over to her. As I approached I could see that she did look a mess but not at death's door.

"I'm going to see you in a little while, Peaches. There are a couple of people here who have appointments and I'll see them first. Briana's going to see you."

"Oh, I met her. She took over from Bobsy."

"That's right. So I'll see you in a bit, OK? Try not to eat all the bagels."

She gave a laugh and nodded.

Olive was standing by the door waiting for me and we went together toward my office. "She sick," I heard her say. Her words seemed odd but I didn't pay attention, really, until, as we got to my office door, Olive said, "Look sick."

"What?" I asked. Olive looked her normal well-dressed, dyed-yellow-hair-in-neat-cornrows self. I followed her into my office and we both sat down.

"Girl, weh rum. Sick."

"Olive, why are you talking like that?"

She looked at me and gave a little shrug and a half smile. "Can talk."

"You can't talk?"

"Neh," she said, shaking her head.

"You can't talk." I said it as a statement. She looked entirely calm and even a little pleased with herself.

"Can talk. Were no come."

"Since when? When did this happen?" Thoughts started flying through my head. A stroke? Encephalitis? Had she had a seizure? Had she been hit in the head?

"Fo. Fo day."

"Four days ago?"

"Yeh."

"This started four days ago and did you tell anyone or go to the emergency room or do anything?"

"Poin. Day," she said, pointing down with her finger.

"Your appointment is today." She nodded as I said this. "You waited until your appointment." She nodded again.

"Is there anything else that's wrong? Have you had a headache or have you felt numb anywhere or lost strength in any of your muscles? Have you had fevers? No seizures, right?" To all of my questions Olive shook her head, gazing at me with clear eyes and an amused look on her face.

"Talk lie baby."

I looked down at the blotter on my desk and gathered my thoughts for a moment. Olive had been taking the protease inhibitor cocktail for several months and her counts hadn't improved as much as I would have liked. In the last few years she'd been coming to appointments with what had become a predictable array of unsubstantiated complaints: the severe abdominal pain that didn't seem to bother her in the waiting room, the frozen shoulder that she moved freely when not focusing on it. The admission for "constant seizures" that found no true seizures at all. I didn't order as many tests as she might have wanted but she did seem to feel better when I acknowledged that she had pain somewhere, or that I understood she was suffering. When she'd come to CSS in the wheelchair after a trip to Hawaii with her mother we didn't order a lot of tests, and after a few weeks she left the wheelchair at home. In 1994 Zoe Prin had taken over Olive's psychiatric care and slowly they explored some of the horrors of Olive's childhood. Sometimes Olive resisted these conversations. She could not make the connection between her psychic pain and her somatic complaints. She could say that she liked being taken care of, but her mind refused to allow her to make the connection with the vast number of times she asked the doctor to address a complaint. I never forgot that Olive had AIDS. Each time she walked in the door with some new problem I first had to rule out HIV or another pathology as the source. As far as this unusual new situation was concerned, I knew of no clinical entity that involved waking up one morning speaking baby talk.

"OK," I said, taking a big breath, "let me examine you. You're also seeing Dr. Prin today, right?" She nodded. I gave her a gown to put on and I went out of the room to let her undress. I walked down the hall to Zoe's office and knocked on her door.

"You aren't going to believe this one." I told her about Olive's newest presentation. She listened with a growing look of surprise and a smile of disbelief on her face. "I'm going to examine her now. I'll send her down to you and let you know what I find."

"OK, thanks. I wonder what's been going on at home. Maybe her mother made another appearance."

"That's a good idea." I remembered when she'd come into the office in the wheelchair after the trip to Hawaii with her mother. Umbrella drinks. "I think I won't ask her about it, though. I'll leave that for you. I think that would be better."

"Yeah, good. I think you're right," she said, nodding. Zoe has bright, expressive brown eyes and thick copper hair that she pulls back into a ponytail. She tucked a stray bit of hair behind her ear. "She's original, I'll give her that."

I did a thorough neurological exam on Olive, noting no findings other than the infantile speech which lessened in the course of the visit. When I commented on this she said, "It come and go." The exam itself, my hands feeling her body and testing her arms and legs, seemed to relieve Olive. I sensed that this act of being examined by her doctor met some of her needs, addressed some of the hurt that she carried so deep inside her. She did not object when I told her that I wanted to wait a while before ordering any CT scans or MRIs.

When I walked out into the hall with Olive, Zoe happened to be bringing another patient back to the waiting room. "Come on with me, Olive, I can see you now."

As they walked away from me I heard Olive say, "Me can talk." And Zoe nodded.

I went back to my office and put my note in the computer as quickly as I could, describing the objective findings and my plan—my plan being not to order a lot of tests and to see what psychiatry suggested. Though tempted, I couldn't just write that my patient was talking like a three-year-old. I had to limit any tendency toward incredulity or sarcasm. Because Olive had a known somatiform disorder I could objectively document my skepticism, but any judgment would not be appropriate. I regarded the chart as a place to communicate with the future. The next doctor or medical student or nurse who happened to be involved with Olive's care would look to the medical record to provide much of his or her information. The chart stood as the record of my actions and decisions, and as a legal document it tended to be dry and impersonal, objective and removed. While it reflected my care, my reasoning, and my decisions, the chart didn't have much room for editorializing and certainly couldn't be used as a place for amusement or inside jokes.

Before computerized medical records I used to be much more colorful in my charts, adding an occasional drawing of a wound or an abscess and sometimes sketching an interesting hat or piece of jewelry. My written charts were also full of doodles. As I chatted with patients or talked on the phone I drew tiny circles, arrows, triangles, and swirls in the margins of any piece of paper in front of me. In residency people used to tell me they would know from opening a patient's chart that I'd been involved in the care because I always somehow left a little striped triangle or a series of circles within circles in the margins of the progress note. At CSS I'd gotten a large paper blotter for my desk and confined my doodling to this surface. Also, since we'd moved from paper charts to computerized records I didn't have the same temptation. The computer standardized many aspects of a patient's record of care but removed some of the idiosyncrasies and what I considered charm of the handwritten chart.

I saw the next patient fairly quickly, a routine visit to check labs and encourage continued compliance with taking the medications. Then I went out to the waiting room to call in Peaches, who had by this time fallen asleep with her head resting on the back of the couch, legs sprawled out in front of her, one hand still clutching a half-eaten bagel. She got up, rubbing her eyes, and followed me back to the hall and my office, carrying her large orange down coat under her arm. She flopped into the armchair in front of my desk and looked up at the ceiling.

"Oh, Dr. Ball, I am definitely dyin'. I know I ain't been comin' to see you and I know you probly think all I been doin' is crack. I won't lie, I did some crack but mostly I been home. Look at my skin." She put the half-eaten bagel on my desk and stuck out her arm, rubbing it vigorously with her hand. The red, irritated skin had a flaky covering and as she rubbed, a shower of fine flakes fell to the carpet. "Oh, sorry," she said, brushing off her arm one last time and pulling down her sleeve. "I been losin' weight like crazy, my mouth is full of that white junk."

"Peaches, it's been nearly a year since you were here. I can't help you if you don't come, if I can't see you to find out what's going on."

"I know, I know. What was my T cells last time?"

"You had a hundred and thirty-four T cells on your last visit—"

"Oh my God, I'm dyin'."

"Well, you don't look like you're dying but I need to examine you and you need to get on some medication. You know we have good medication now, it's really helping people."

"Not AZT."

"No, I won't try to get you to take AZT."

"Well, I'll take whatever you got. I got to."

"OK, first let me do your exam and we'll do some blood tests today." I got up and gave her a gown to change into. Peaches sat quietly on my examining table while I took her blood pressure and checked out her eyes and ears and the thrush in her mouth. I felt the lymph nodes in her neck and listened to her heart and lungs. She lay on her back and I examined her breasts and abdomen, felt her legs and ankles. The same flaky red skin on her arms covered most of her back and face as well. As I washed my hands I asked, "Did you talk to Briana? Are the boys OK?"

"Sheesh, yeah, driving me crazy, bunch a wild things." She smiled.

"How old is your youngest now?"

"Tyrell's eleven. He's the worst of them." She gave a short laugh and scratched her arm, creating another little shower of flaking skin. "Spoiled as shit, that one."

I laughed. "OK, get dressed and I'll give you some prescriptions before you go down to the nurses for your blood work." As I stepped out into the hall to let her change, Katie approached me from her office.

"Susan, I just was talking to one of the social workers at New Hope House and she asked if I knew a patient named Marco."

"Marco Prava?" I asked.

"Yes, him. She knew that he'd been a patient here before and apparently he died there quite a while ago, but she wanted to tell me that they have another patient there now who happens to be Marco's cousin. She said Marco's mother comes to visit him sometimes."

I knew that Marco had died. His mother had finally agreed to place him in a nursing home after he'd been at home for a week with his terrible diarrhea and she'd had to change his bed more times than she could count. Not surprisingly, she practically lived at the nursing home herself for the few more weeks that Marco spent there. I remembered Mrs. Prava sitting in the dark hospital room next to her son's empty bed while he was off at a test, telling me that she knew he had AIDS. It seemed so long ago.

"Wow, that was about two years ago I think. He had horrible cryptosporidium. What a nice guy and the mother was so devoted to him. How sad for her to have to be back in that place."

"Yeah, the social worker said she's very nice. Sad, though. Anyway, I was just talking to her about another patient and she mentioned this and then here you were in the hall."

Katie started working at CSS in early 1996. She didn't know Marco or his mother and she had not been around for very long before the protease inhibitors came out. I wondered if she could imagine what I meant when I spoke of horrible cryptosporidium. Her reference points for AIDS patients would be so different without the history of those long years when there wasn't any effective treatment.

I went back into my office where Peaches sat eating the rest of her bagel. "So, let's do this for today, Peaches. I'm going to give you some fluconazole for the thrush in your mouth and a pill so you don't get PCP. I'm going to give you some mild lotion for that rash but I'll make you an appointment to see the dermatologist later this week."

"Damn rash, what a mess, my bed is full of dead skin."

I could only imagine. I didn't want to. "So the next thing is the medication for the HIV. There are three prescriptions, three medications that you'll get. The first one, indinavir, you have to take three times a day, that's every eight hours, and you have to take it on an empty stomach. So you wake up at eight, say, and take it and wait an hour before you eat breakfast. Then you need to take it at four p.m. and then at midnight, each time without eating for two hours before the medication and one hour after. I'm also giving you stavudine, which you take twice a day, and lamivudine twice a day." As the words came out of my mouth, I wondered how in the world someone as disorganized as Peaches could possibly follow such instructions. Most people couldn't. I must be insane. "I'm going to write it all down for you, OK? And I want you to call me if you have any questions or any problems with it."

She was looking at me skeptically. "Dr. Ball, that sounds like a lot of pills."

"It is. You're right. It's a lot of pills."

"Can't you just give me one pill?"

I smiled at her. "I know, right? That would be the best thing. But I can't. All the pills do different things and you need to get your T cells up. The medicine works, we know it does."

"Well I'm dyin' so it damn well better work." She watched as I wrote prescription after prescription and handed them to her one after another, the little pile of papers growing in her hand.

When I finished I went over the instructions with her once more. I had her read what I'd written. Once or twice before I'd been surprised when a patient could not read. It always made me think of Maggie and her illiterate boyfriend, only less exotic or happy. Peaches read my instructions without a problem although toward the end of the list her eyebrows rose up in her face and she gave one of those belly laughs of hers. "I sure hope these pills is small because there sure is a damn lot of 'em."

I felt hopeful as I watched her walk down the hall to the lab to get her blood drawn. Her T cells would go up and her skin would clear. Her thrush would resolve. She'd get off crack and her boys would graduate from high school. These things could happen, all of them.

Later, in clinic rounds, the day's patients were presented. Many patients at CSS were now taking cocktails of protease inhibitors. Many struggled with side effects, stopping the regimen within days of starting, complaining of upset stomachs or just too many pills. Some patients resisted taking anything at all, ever wary of the myths from the earlier days of AZT, claiming a friend started taking medication and promptly died. I wondered if that thought might be lurking somewhere in Sabir's mind. Maybe his reason for refusing everything wasn't so much an unwillingness to engage with his own illness; maybe he was afraid because of something that had happened to someone else. Maybe he knew someone who died after starting meds.

When Sabir's name was called I presented his case and admitted my frustration with getting him to accept any treatments. I wondered out loud if maybe he had a friend who'd had a bad experience, but Paul Ferand shook his head. "No, I asked him the same thing today. He actually knows someone who is doing quite well. He's stuck for now in his inability to face what's happening to him, despite all the physical changes." Oh well, I thought. So much for that idea.

Olive's latest set of symptoms met with more than a few rolled eyes around the table. What better way to get attention than to speak baby talk? Zoe reported that there had recently been another interaction between the patient and her mother, and that Olive's coping skills became overwhelmed at these encounters. We decided not to pursue further imaging tests at this time; we'd stay in close touch with her and offer support through this episode. I shook my head, amazed at the innate creativity that Olive's conversion reaction implied. She didn't sit down and ask herself how she could deal with her feelings; her feelings just took over. Gerald looked at me and said, "You can't make this stuff up."

When I finally presented Peaches at the end of rounds I voiced my concern with her advanced disease and my doubts that she could take all those medications.

"She'll be back, don't worry," said Stan.

"Well, I guess that would be a start, at this point," I acknowledged; at least she might come and see us a little more often.

"She swears a lot at her kids," said Briana. "One of them called her while she was in my office and she must have used the f-bomb five or six times in one sentence!"

"What she lacks in vocabulary she more than makes up for in enthusiasm," I said, smiling. "I just hope that she'll be as enthusiastic about her medications."

# Chapter Fifteen

# 1997 Amazing Changes

When I saw her name on my schedule in February 1997 I envisioned a small, dark-skinned woman with very pink gums, no teeth, and an enormous line of sutures marching across her forehead under a maroon knit cap. Pregnant Pat who wanted an apartment. I remembered seeing her once, some eight or nine months later, how she dismissively answered my questions about her pregnancy with a wave of her hand. "Oh, it died," she said, rooting around in her purse among the keys, crumpled cigarette packages, candy wrappers, and ancient-looking pieces of mail. After that visit she'd disappeared, missing the next several appointments, and eventually her name stopped appearing on my schedule altogether. Until today, that is.

The woman who walked into my office when I called Pat's name did not resemble that earlier memory except for the small, dark-skinned part. This woman had her hair neatly pulled back and wore a clean black winter coat over a yellow blouse and navy slacks. She wore comfortable-looking black lace-up shoes with black rubber soles. This woman had a brilliant smile accentuated by a set of gleaming white dentures. "How you doin', Dr. Ball?" she said, sitting down in the chair in front of my desk as I looked at her in amazement.

"Pat? It's really you?"

"Why you lookin' at me like that? I ain't dead yet!" and she laughed, the teeth practically sparkling in her mouth.

"Pat, you look fantastic. Teeth and everything. Where've you been?"

"I spent some time on the island."

"Long Island?"

"Rikers."

"Oh," I said. I hadn't ever heard the prison on Rikers Island referred to as if it were a summer vacation spot. Stan would love that. "So it looks like they took pretty good care of you there."

"Yeah, I got my teeth finally an' they gave me my medications every day. I need refills, though. They only gave me a few days when I left."

"Do you know the medications you're taking?"

"Vira-something, I take one pill two times a day, and I take Combivir. You gave me that before but I never took it. They did my T cells last week and they was four hundred and twenty-two." She positively beamed as she relayed this news, resembling nothing like the sex-for-drugs shambles that she'd been two years ago.

"That's awesome. How great. I can order the refills for you. Where are you now? Where are you living?"

"I'm goin' to my mother's house in Pennsylvania."

"Today? You're living there now?"

"I been in the hotel since I got out but I ain't gonna stay there. Once I get my 'scriptions I'm goin' to Philly."

"And have you been clean since you got out?"

"Hell, yeah. I ain't goin' back to Rikers no time soon."

She rummaged in her purse—I saw the inevitable cigarettes—and she found the prison medical papers that they'd given her on the day she was released. We went through her list of medications and I read that she'd been on effective HIV therapy for over a year, her T cell counts rising steadily. Pat reported that she'd gone every day to the dispensary where the nurses gave her the pills. She said that lots of inmates lined up to take medications, whereas they used to be suspicious or wary of the ineffective regimens previously doled out by the prison authorities. Even the HIV-infected prison population knew about successful treatment of the virus.

After I examined Pat, the scar from her distant misadventure with the knife-wielding sex-for-drugs partner now a thin pink wrinkle across her forehead, I noted what prescriptions she'd need before I sent her down to the lab to have her blood drawn. In addition to the list on the sheet from Rikers, she said she had to have two asthma inhalers, a brand-name anti-inflammatory drug for muscle aches, another brand-name medication for allergies, and two different sleeping pills. It sounded as if she was stocking her street-drug pharmacy. All of these medications had value for someone wishing to sell them instead of take them. Sell them and turn around to spend the money on crack. Painkillers and narcotics usually topped the list but I guessed Pat had too much savvy to ask me for those. As she rattled off her wish list I realized that it was going to take more than a year in jail and a new set of teeth to make Pat into a different person.

I tried to put it to her gently. "Pat, listen, you haven't been on any of these things for the last year and this is your first time seeing me in a very long time. I'm not going to prescribe other medicines for you today. I am thrilled to see you looking so well and you seem happy, too. Let's not add anything at all right now."

She started to protest as I talked, but I held up my hand to stop her and finished what I had to say. Somewhere it seemed to occur to her that she liked the way she felt. Maybe she didn't need to go back to her old life, at least not just yet. I gave myself a mental high five when she closed her purse and nodded. OK, I didn't need to write those other prescriptions. Still, I hoped that her mother's house in Philadelphia was in a good neighborhood and not full of drugs and crack dealers.

Pat's recovery looked beautiful to me, her life's potential vastly different from what it had been a few short years ago. But oh so fragile, I could see. Jail offered structure and support, regularly dispensed medications and trips to the dentist. Pat's framework for survival on her own, learned from years on the street, coming from the most basic and self-degrading list of options, did not include such structure. I thought of my patient Brian, a severe and desperate intravenous drug addict who had turned his life around entirely when he received his HIV test results. He'd gone back to school and now had a job he really liked. He took great care of himself and reached out to others to help them get off drugs. If I could write a prescription for that sense of self-worth and determination I would order a double dose for Pat. Instead I sent her to get her blood drawn, offering words of encouragement and praise which I know she heard but which I'm afraid dissolved too quickly in the air between us.

As I watched Pat walk down the hall away from me, Molly came out of her office and nearly bumped into her.

"Whoa, sorry," she said and backed up. "Oh my gosh. Pat? Is that you? Whoa baby, that smile is blinding!" They walked on down the hall together.

Etta came next. Often her son Joey came with her and stood silently in front of my desk playing with paper clips as his mother and I spoke over his head, but today Etta came in alone. This would be the third time I'd seen her since her hospitalization last summer.

"Dr. Ball, why do you want me to come every six weeks? I take two subways and a bus to get here and nothing is any different. What's the point?"

"Hi, Etta, you're looking great. How are you feeling?"

She gave me one of her sneers and dramatically sighed. "I'm fine."

"I've wanted you to come in so we can keep track of you and monitor the meds and make sure you are getting what you need. You've missed a few appointments since last summer so it isn't really even close to every six weeks."

"I told you I'm taking everything. What do you need to see me for?"

"How are you feeling?"

"I'm fine. I said I'm fine."

"Yes, you did, sorry to ask the same question." I looked at her sheet and saw that she'd gained another eight pounds since her last visit. "Etta, what's your baseline weight? How much did you weigh, say, three or four years ago, before you got sick?"

She looked at the ceiling, thinking, chewing her gum. I noticed the eyeliner, mascara, and lipstick; she'd started wearing makeup again after a few months out of the hospital. "I used to always weigh one eighty-five. That was my regular weight."

"And how tall are you?"

"Five two."

"Last summer, when you were sick, your weight was down to a hundred and twenty-two and then you probably even lost a few more pounds when you were hospitalized. And now you're back up to a hundred and sixty. You're a good weight now. Even a bit heavy for how tall you are."

"Yeah, well, I'm going to be gaining some more."

"Do you want to see the nutritionist? So you don't get too heavy?"

"No."

"I know you're used to being heavier but one sixty is plenty for your height, and being heavy puts you at risk for other medical problems, things like high blood pressure and diabetes."

She looked up at the ceiling again, jaw working her gum. She appeared to be thinking about something so I just watched her for a moment. No woman can be too thin or too rich, I thought. Who said that? Probably someone thin and rich. I'd been brought up in a culture where this statement could have been posted above all the doorways and driveways. Popular white media drove a strong message of thin waists and long, slender legs for women, the latter being a stretch from my own personal reality but a wistful mirage nonetheless. For many of my female patients, however, their culture encouraged a significantly larger version of this ideal. More than once I'd been told as I walked down the hall, "Dr. Ball, you put on some weight, you lookin' good!" to my mortification. Etta's zaftig form looked ample enough to me. I had a hard time understanding why she'd want to gain still more weight.

"I'm pregnant," she said, looking bored.

It took a moment for that to register. Well, I thought, so much for my cultural competence. I had a brief mental picture of grabbing my computer keyboard, picking it up, and smashing it down on my desk. A rush of thoughts blasted rapid-fire through my head, most of them angry and exasperated. She's pregnant. She's less than nine months off her deathbed, it's been arduous to get her to take her meds, she resists coming to the doctor, she makes me mad. A few random swear words were sprinkled here and there as well.

"I must say, you surprised me with that one," I managed, calmly.

"Yeah, well."

"I remember two years ago, when I was pregnant with my son, and you said you wanted another baby. Are you feeling OK? Do you want to keep the pregnancy?"

"Yeah. I wasn't trying to get pregnant but I'm going to keep it."

"Are you involved with the father?"

She made a dismissive, waving motion with her hand and shook her head. "No."

"Does he know that you're pregnant?"

"Oh, I don't know. It's possible. No, probably not. Maybe. I don't know."

I realized that my eyebrows had been lifting steadily as she spoke. I tried to bring them down to a less questioning level. "Do you know who the father is?"

"Well, I know there's more than one possibility. But probably it's this one guy. And no, he probably doesn't know. I just met him in the bar."

"What about the HIV?"

"What?"

"Do you let your partners know? Do you try to get them to use condoms?"

Again the wave of the hand and a sneering, *tsk*ing noise came from her. "We don't talk about that."

"And will you tell this guy? About the pregnancy? About the HIV?"

"It's none of his business, really. I'm not interested in that guy. What I want to know is if I should stop the medication since I'm pregnant. I didn't take it for the last two weeks."

This was going from bad to worse. Now I wanted to stand up and scream. But I didn't, instead saying, in what I hoped was a quiet, reasonable tone of voice, "Um, Etta, please don't do that. I wish you had called or something. Remember, we've talked every time about not stopping the medication?"

"Yeah, well I wasn't pregnant then. I am now. These medicines might be poison, who knows?"

"You're absolutely right to be cautious and I'm glad that at least you are telling me about it now. Your regimen is a good one and we don't know of any side effects that jeopardize the pregnancy or birth defects associated with the medications that you're taking. What's very important, though, is that you keep your viral load suppressed so that the HIV doesn't get transmitted to the baby. I strongly urge you to get back on the medication today. And not stop it. Can I make you an OB appointment?"

"No, I went already. In Queens. It's closer to my house."

"You told them about the HIV, right?"

"Well, not exactly. They do the test so they're gonna know about it anyway."

"Yes. That's true." I found myself taking deep breaths. "I can give you a list of your meds to give to them so they'll know that you're getting your care here, and what your counts have been."

"Yeah, OK."

"OK, great. Let me do your exam and then I'll write a note for you."

After her exam and the note, she went down to the lab and I stood by the big window behind my desk. I could see the East River and the Triboro Bridge in the distance. I could see York Avenue twenty-four stories below and the cars moving slowly in both directions. Years later a small airplane was going to smash into the brick apartment building just one block to the north, in whose windows I could now make out curtains and lamps.

I didn't know where to put Etta's pregnancy in my mind. Last summer, after all those years of careless refusal, she'd unexpectedly taken the pills that I prescribed after her hospitalization. Within two months her health improved and she gained weight. She reported never skipping a dose of medication. She put on makeup and looked great. I felt glad for her and glad for her little son, Joey, who would not lose his mother as it had seemed he so surely would. Perhaps I shouldn't have been surprised to hear that she'd been going out to bars and having sex again. Why did I think that healthy Etta on effective medication would somehow be different from healthy Etta pre-HIV? When I tried to emphasize the importance of condoms she gave me her trademark sneer. This pregnancy seemed like a bad idea for so many reasons. I wished she'd given herself a little longer to be well and stable. I couldn't know at the time that I wouldn't see Etta again for nearly two years.

Patients felt comfortable in our big waiting room with its upholstered chairs and couches. A large bouquet of flowers arrived every week through a generous donation to our clinic: lilies, roses, tulips, and birds of paradise all meticulously arranged in a vase in the middle of the room. I doubt there are many HIV clinics that have fresh flowers in the waiting room. I was thinking about this as I stood at the elevators later that afternoon, on my way down to the inpatient floor. I looked at the stargazer lilies; they reminded me of exuberant red and white horns, as if they'd play trumpet concertos if they could. Then the elevator doors opened and a guy who looked like a handsome, tough street kid pushed out a small young woman whose hands gripped the arms of her wheelchair. I stepped back to let them pass and the man said, "Hey, Dr. Ball." The woman looked up at me and smiled.

I blinked to make sure my eyes were not tricking me. "Oh my God. I can't believe it."

"Hi, Dr. Ball," she said, in that nasal voice of hers.

"Sabitha, oh my gosh, look at you!" Alive. I didn't say it but I certainly thought it. We'd sent her to a nursing home over a year ago. She'd been close to the bottom of her downward-spiraling course and I did not expect ever to see her again. As I'd watched them leaving together that day, I'd wondered what could possibly happen to her four kids, knowing that Sabitha's mother drank too much and the boyfriend was not the father of the children. Their mother was going to a skilled nursing facility because she couldn't walk or feed herself and in all likelihood would die in a matter of weeks. But no, here she was, back in our waiting room. Still in a wheelchair but smiling and talking and alive!

"What a great surprise this is to see you! To see you both."

"She got home from Plainview last week. We're here to see the social worker," said the boyfriend, looking happy.

Sabitha continued to smile up at me.

"Are you back at home now?" When she nodded I asked, "Did they give you the new medications at Plainview?"

"Yeah. A lot of pills. But I took 'em all."

"Did they give you pills to go home with? Do you need prescriptions?" I directed the question to the boyfriend, whose name I could not recall.

"She has enough until we see you. She's got an appointment with you next week. We're just seeing the social worker today." He still looked like a teenager with his big diamond in one ear and the black baseball cap. If I saw the guy on the street I wouldn't imagine he was the type of person to stay with a girlfriend while she lived for a year in a nursing home and nearly died of AIDS. Looking more closely, I saw that his eyes had a faint weariness about them.

I reached out and put my hand on his arm. "Thank you for bringing her back. I'll see you then. Sabitha, keep taking those pills. I'll see you next week."

"I will." Her voice sounded like someone was squeezing her from behind and her head bobbed as she spoke. I could see that while she'd recovered a good deal from her severe neurological deterioration, certain deficits persisted.

Her boyfriend pushed her over to the front desk to check in for their appointment. What a wonderful surprise to see Sabitha alive!

The elevator door opened again and Stewart came off, an hour early for his appointment with me. Before he said anything I assured him that I'd be back upstairs in a short while and he had other appointments before mine. He looked worriedly after me as the elevator door shut between us.

When I returned I got off the elevator on the twenty-third floor and went up the back way to my office. This avoided a trip through the waiting room and the possibility of spontaneously bumping into Stewart again. Walking through the waiting room could be very costly on a busy day, as patients inevitably corralled me as I went by. "Dr. Ball, I need a letter to get a new mattress." "Dr. Ball, can you please rewrite that cough medicine prescription you gave me last year?" "Dr. Ball, I've got a very dry mouth and every time I swallow I can taste phlegm in my throat. Can you see me today? Just for a minute?" I hated saying no, but interruptions had the potential to sabotage a day. I could keep on schedule only if these requests went through the front desk.

I got back to my office and looked through Stewart's chart before calling him in. Twice in the past he'd had clots in his leg. Now he took blood thinners daily and we regularly checked a blood test to monitor the level of anticoagulation. It had been a major project to get him on this medication when he'd been hospitalized the first time. He asked me about forty-five thousand times if he really needed to take it. Nothing I said seemed to get through to him. Finally one day the patient in the bed next to his, after hearing our conversation for the third day in a row, yelled over, "Stewart, take the damn Coumadin. My wife takes it." So he did. I didn't ask why. I just felt enormously relieved that I could stop talking to him about it.

Now we'd moved on to the next therapeutic decision. Stewart had a fragile immune system and I wanted him to take a protease inhibitor, but each time I addressed the issue we'd go around in the same circles. He worried about having AIDS and the fact that his counts remained low, but his anxiety always led him to say no when I suggested he take an additional medication. Instead Stewart took yoga and meditation classes and he insisted on my prescribing him a slew of vitamins, all in an effort to treat his HIV through what he called "alternative" means. I didn't object to any of this and encouraged him to do as much meditation and yoga as he could; anything to ease his anxiety. He just wouldn't take the medication that I knew would help him the most.

As I went out to call him in for his appointment I steeled myself for another frustrating session. I'd ask him about improving his antiretroviral regimen and he'd ask me if he really needed to, if the medication had toxicity, if people were allergic to it, if I could prescribe a lower dose than recommended. He asked good questions but he didn't listen to the answers. Instead he repeated the questions. I could try to rephrase my responses but that never really helped. Sometimes I asked him, "Stewart, why do you ask the same questions if you want me to give you a different answer?" I don't think he understood my point. I often felt like I'd failed in some way, not being able to ease his mind or overcome his resistance to my suggestions. I wanted to help him get better, yet I couldn't seem to do it. I went to the door of the waiting room and waved at him to come in.

As soon as he sat down in my office Stewart said, "I think I should start taking indinavir, don't you think?"

I sat there for a moment looking at him with my mouth half-open. Stewart's personality could not have led him to say this as a joke, but I wondered if he might be kidding just to irritate me. The idea flickered there in my brain for an instant and I saw myself jumping up from my chair and flinging my arms up over my head and screaming as loudly as I could. I had to give a little shake and clear my throat.

"Stewart, is that really *you* saying that? You aren't someone disguised as Stewart trying to pull my leg?"

"No, Dr. Ball, it's me. I just think, you know, I've heard some really good things about indinavir and don't you think it would be a good idea for me to take it?"

"I've been trying for months and months to convince you."

"Well, I know," he said, wiping his hand across his brow, pushing back the thin wisps of his hair so they lay down in long strands. "I read a story in the paper where a guy with AIDS had his T cell count go back up to six hundred when he was taking indinavir."

"That's great, Stewart, that's a great story. You know, he's not the only one."

"Will my T cells go up to six hundred if I take indinavir?"

"I don't have a crystal ball. I can't tell you if they'll go back up that high. But I will tell you that your T cells are definitely *not* going to go up unless you start taking some better medications."

"How high will they go?"

I couldn't answer this. "I'm so glad that you're ready to start taking it. It's a great decision on your part and I'm so glad that you read that article. I'd like you to take stavudine as well, to be on a cocktail. I don't want to start you on indinavir alone. The guy in your article wasn't just taking indinavir."

"No, I just want the indinavir. I'm already on Combivir. I'll keep taking what I'm on and start it. That's two. That's enough."

An effective regimen involved three drugs, one protease inhibitor and two drugs from the AZT class known as reverse-transcriptase inhibitors. Stewart was on two drugs in this latter class already, in a combination pill that he took twice a day. Two years ago I'd almost gotten him to take the new saquinavir but he backed out after he'd brought up the subject himself. I feared that the virus had become resistant to the two-drug regimen he was taking now. Adding just one new drug at a time didn't seem like a good idea, but I didn't want to push him too hard because he might change his mind about the indinavir as well.

"OK, it's not optimal but it would be great for you to be on indinavir. I'm glad you want to give it a try."

"I won't get any side effects, will I?" His eyebrows rose up and his forehead had three deep furrows.

"We've been over this, you know. We've talked about this many, many times. It's a drug that needs to be taken on an empty stomach and it might make you feel queasy in the first days that you're on it. Most people do fine. It would never have gotten approved if the side effects made it impossible to tolerate. And it doesn't have sulfa, it's not like Bactrim, which I'm guessing is your next question."

"No sulfa?"

"No." Now I wondered if I'd shot myself in the foot, bringing up his dreaded issue of drug allergies and the fact that Bactrim had nearly killed him before he became my patient. He would inevitably ask this question, so maybe I just saved some time. Or not.

"If I take it on an empty stomach does that mean no food?"

Sometimes he could really make me wonder. I nodded. "It means you wait two hours to take it after you've eaten a meal and you wait an hour to eat after you take it. And it's every eight hours. It's not like other drugs that are taken three times a day where you take one in the morning, one at noontime, and one in the evening. This really needs to be every eight hours. So that means eight a.m., four p.m., and midnight. Or some combination like that. Do you think you can do that?"

"Gee, Dr. Ball, I don't know. Three times a day. That seems like a lot. Don't you think twice a day is enough? These are strong medicines. That guy's T cells went up to six hundred."

"Yes and that's because he took his indinavir every eight hours."

"Yeah, it did say something about that, about adjusting to taking the medicine that way." Stewart had both his hands on the knees of his blue jeans, nodding as he hunched his shoulders.

"You're going to do great on this, Stewart. You are a very organized guy and once you make up your mind about something you're very consistent. Once you get started, you'll see it's something you can do."

"Oh, I don't know . . ."

*Aargh*, I thought, *don't let him get away!*

"Here's the prescription," I said, writing quickly, signing my name, and tearing it off the pad. "Let me examine you now and then go read that article again. Jean will meet with you before you leave to go over all the things I've said, and if you have more questions she'll answer them or come and ask me. We'll do your labs today and then again in four to six weeks. Stewart, your viral load is going to go down and your CD4 count is going to go up. You'll be happy when you see that happen."

He nodded as I said that. "Really? You really think so?"

"If you take it correctly I'm sure that will happen." I got up and washed my hands at the sink and took out my stethoscope as he went to sit on the examining table.

Later on in rounds I sat next to Felicity. "I don't know how you did it, my dear," she said. "Stewart told me that he is going to start taking indinavir." Her hair always gradually fell out of its loose bun in the course of the day, but never did she look anything less than elegant. As Stewart's social worker she'd heard a lot of his stories over the years. Stewart took advantage of her endless patience but she never said anything harsh about him. She and I often compared notes at the end of a clinic day when we'd both seen him. I'd be vocal with my frustrations and she'd merely sigh and say, "Oh yes, I know, he can be so worried." I don't think Stewart knew how fortunate he was.

As we slowly went through the list of patients seen at CSS that day, Stewart's name came up early. I looked over at Stan as I revealed that Stewart had finally agreed to take a protease inhibitor but would be starting only one new drug, continuing his previous Combivir, which he'd been taking for over a year. Stan shrugged with a resigned look.

"I know." I nodded.

"But, shit, it's about time he took *something*." Stan had covered Stewart more than a few times over the years and he had heard my presentations at rounds when I'd been unable to get Stewart to take effective therapy. Stan had a couple of patients with personalities to rival Stewart's so he knew what I was up against. The new regimen for Stewart would not be optimal and we both knew it. I held up crossed fingers.

We continued through the list.

Gerald called Sabitha's name and I shook my head, saying, "Today had some surprises and this was one of them. She didn't have an appointment with me but I nearly fell over when she came off the elevator. She's still in a wheelchair but I just couldn't believe it. We sent her to a nursing home a year ago."

"Sabitha? *That* Sabitha?" asked Dan. "I covered her one weekend; the one with the bad encephalopathy? She's not dead?"

"She is not dead. And her same boyfriend was pushing the wheelchair. That was really something"

"I didn't know her from before," said Katie, the social worker now assigned to Sabitha's case. "She and the boyfriend came to go over her benefits and make the changes now that she's actually out of the nursing home, back at her mother's house. The kids have been living there too; it's a bit tight even though the apartment's got three bedrooms. Her benefits are not in bad shape as the mother gets SSI. I called the Medicaid office and they have the right information to get Sabitha back on public assistance. Her boyfriend said the kids are a bit wild. I'll follow up and see her again next week when she comes to see you," she said, looking over at me.

"Great, thanks." I shook my head again, smiling.

On we went through the list. I presented Etta and the troubling news of her pregnancy. Molly said that she'd pressed for a little more information about the father of the baby but Etta had not wanted to talk about him at all. "She looks great," said Molly, "but looking great seems to have gotten her right back to where she started." Molly said she'd give Etta a call in a few weeks to make sure she was getting prenatal care.

Gerald called out the next patient, someone Dan took care of. And then he spoke Pat's name. "Talk about coming back from the dead," commented Molly wryly.

"Jiminy Cricket, today was wild," I said, to begin. "So, I last saw Pat more than two years ago, shortly after she'd miscarried, which was shortly after she'd had her forehead sliced open as she was trading sex for drugs."

"Guess she had an unhappy customer," observed Stan.

"Stop that," came from Molly.

"She came in today looking like a totally new woman. She's on meds, she's clean, she had nice clothes and she had teeth."

"Oh my God, the teeth!" Molly wore a disbelieving smile.

"It was another amazing surprise in my day today. She looked fantastic. So I asked her where she'd been. And she said she'd been on the island."

Stan hooted with laughter. "And I'll bet she didn't mean Nantucket!"

"You've got that one right," I said.

# Chapter Sixteen

# 1999  Despite Our Best Intentions

We had effective therapy to treat HIV. It worked. The medication suppressed viral replication, viral loads went down, and T cells went up. Better immune function meant that patients were less apt to get sick, less apt to die. But almost as soon as we happily saw that patients on highly active antiretroviral therapy—HAART, as we called it at the time—did well, we realized that patients who missed doses ran into problems. Sporadic adherence resulted in fluctuating drug levels and allowed virus to escape. If patients skipped doses or forgot them or took the weekend off too many times, their viral loads became once again detectable. In the presence of subtherapeutic drug levels, canny HIV adjusted itself, altering its genetic makeup to become resistant to one or more of the medications in the regimen. A virus resistant to a medication could not be suppressed on the same regimen, so the medication had to be switched. Frequently the genetic mutation of the virus that resulted in resistance also made the virus resistant to other medications in the same class. So even though the patient had never taken a drug called Z in the protease inhibitor class, he or she might, in fact, be resistant to Z because of resistance to another protease inhibitor. This resulted in restricting our choices for the next drug regimen.

Norbert got very mad at me one day when I told him that his virus demonstrated resistance to drugs X, Y, and Z along with drugs A, B, and C. "How could I possibly be resistant to Z?" he asked. "I've never taken Z for even one day." He shook his head disgustedly, all but saying, "How did I get such a stupid doctor?"

"I know that it doesn't seem right," I said, nodding my head, "but we call this cross-resistance because Z is in the same class of drugs as X and Y. HIV is a very smart virus."

Norbert sat across from me with folded arms, his shoulder muscles bulging in his tight dark turtleneck. He had close-cut black hair and smooth, dark skin. "That's just crazy," he said, in his lilting Jamaican accent. He gave a characteristic sniff and shook his head again.

Norbert didn't like to take the medication for HIV. The burden of it became my fault and he blamed me for his viral load rising, saying I prescribed too many pills. "Why can't you give me one pill? I could take one pill, but, Dr. Ball, you want me to take pills all day, every day, and that's just impossible." He didn't mind taking pills for allergies or headaches or antibiotics if he had a cold, but the everyday, weeks and months on end, nature of treating his HIV rattled him. He missed doses frequently. At every visit we talked of it and the nurses met with him to reinforce the importance of staying consistent in order to keep his virus suppressed. But taking pills bugged him: a constant reminder of an illness that he didn't see or feel, an illness that he hated. And because his drug levels weren't steady, his virus became resistant. By 1999 he'd started and stopped four different HAART regimens and only one or two drugs on our list would now have any suppressive effect at all.

We all knew that treating HIV involved taking a lot of pills, overcoming the many potential side effects, and dealing with the possible toxicity of long-term treatment. Norbert and patients like him resented their HIV and the medication to treat it. He had a lot of company in this regard. In my training and in my career we had always used the term "noncompliance" when we spoke of patients who didn't take their medications or who repeatedly missed appointments. The word implies a lack of obedience. But the reasons why patients couldn't or wouldn't take their medications as prescribed were as numerous as the colors in an autumn sunset, and the patronizing connotations of "compliance" grated on both providers and patients. In recognition of this fact, in AIDS care we began referring to patients' "adherence" rather than their "compliance." Because so many patients struggled to take their pills, "nonadherence" seemed more realistic.

Norbert told me the truth about how often he skipped his medications. I appreciated his honesty, sympathizing with his wish for something simpler. Too often patients lied about taking their pills. They didn't want to disappoint me or they didn't want to hear—again—about the importance of adherence. Their lab tests didn't lie, however. I could usually tell from the results if a patient had been honest or not. If the viral load didn't budge I knew that the patient hadn't taken the medicine. If the viral load became suppressed but then started rising again I could be fairly sure that too many doses were being missed. On the one hand, the lab results helped me; they couldn't prevaricate. But on the other, I never enjoyed having a confrontation with a patient when the test results contradicted what the patient told me.

I wondered sometimes if Norbert snorted a lot of cocaine because he always seemed to have the sniffles. He didn't work and he didn't go to school. Sometime in the past, before he'd started coming to CSS, he'd gotten pneumonia and a doctor had signed papers that qualified him as disabled. Now he collected a check from the disability office every month and spent a lot of time at the gym. He admitted to me that he felt frustrated and bored. I often encouraged him to try to get back into the workforce. He reasoned that whatever job he got would cause him to lose both the government medical insurance and the disability money. He barely scraped by on this money but he didn't want the hassle of all the paperwork. His hollow excuses reverberated beneath his lack of motivation.

In March 1999 he came to the office to show me a painless raised spot on his penis, a round open wound the size of a quarter. Norbert had syphilis. I sent him for a blood test to be sure and gave him an appointment to return the next day for treatment. The results came back positive. He got his shots and came into my office.

"I had syphilis once before," he said, sitting down. "I didn't think I could get it a second time."

"Sad but true. There's a lot of it out there, unfortunately."

"Great." He looked annoyed.

"Did you let your partner know?"

He shook his head, not meeting my eyes.

"Listen, Norbert, it's your decision whether you take your medication or not. Ultimately, if your T cells go down because your viral load is not suppressed it's you who will be dealing with the possibility of getting sick. But syphilis to me means that you're not using condoms. This is dangerous for others and it's not OK. Someone gave you syphilis. You could say that they weren't protecting you. Possibly they didn't know they had it. Who knows? The thing is, you don't have just HIV now. You have resistant HIV. If you infect someone else with your HIV they might do fine.

You seem fine, I know. But your HIV in another person might be a much more aggressive virus, might make them much sicker much more quickly. And it's resistant to a number of medications which makes it that much harder to treat. I'm telling you all of this because you need to be more responsible."

"It's at the club. Most everyone has it already," he said, interrupting me.

"But you have a very resistant virus. The point is, if you pass that to someone else they're going to have resistant virus as well. A highly resistant virus could be catastrophic for another person. Do you understand what I'm saying to you?"

"I need to use condoms."

"You need to use condoms."

He sighed. He looked over at the bulletin board near my desk. "It's just so frustrating, Dr. Ball. You have no idea what a drag it is to have this disease."

I sat at my desk in front of him and wondered what to say. I thought of all the people dying from AIDS and how, looking at Norbert, no one would ever guess he had the infection. He worked out, he stayed in shape. He wore a new shirt with a Ralph Lauren logo and clean dark jeans. When I first met him five years ago, I had nothing to offer him to treat his HIV and I could predict a grim story. Now things had changed. He didn't need to be on disability and yet he wouldn't or couldn't get himself off it. And condoms for him served only as a reminder of a condition he wanted to forget.

"Norbert, I've seen a lot of people die from this illness. We have good medicine now and it works well. But you see what this is like for you. I just don't want to have you infect someone else."

"I know," he said. "I know."

"And your virus now is a particularly dangerous one because it's so resistant. It's very important that you keep this in mind." I stood up to walk him out, gesturing to the fishbowl full of condoms that sits on the counter next to the sink. All of the offices and the front desk at CSS keep condoms available. "Help yourself," I told Norbert. "For now, I'm not suggesting you change regimens again. Not yet anyway, because I don't have a good regimen to put you on. A newer protease is coming out soon and we'll talk about getting you on it. Try not to miss any doses in the meantime, OK?"

Norbert nodded, taking a few condoms as he left.

As I sat back down at my desk I wondered about the public health implications of all the people like Norbert out there going to clubs and having unprotected sex with each other. The gay community had been heroic in its activism and organization in the late 1980s and early 1990s. Their efforts were directly responsible for galvanizing Congress and drug companies into action to get funding and find quicker pathways for approval of HIV treatments. So it puzzled me that gay men would put one another at risk. I once heard Larry Kramer, a great playwright and vocal AIDS activist, speak. His passion and intensity moved everyone in the large auditorium. He chastised the gay community for being too lax with their sexuality and too thoughtless of the dire consequences of their sexual appetites. Norbert didn't want to think about HIV or consequences. I couldn't be his conscience but somehow I had to help him see his role in the epidemic.

Unlike Norbert, Sophia took her medication. She didn't miss her CSS appointments and routinely showed up with some cleavage-revealing, overly tight shirt and very heavy mascara. In the summer it seemed she hardly wore anything at all, the rose tattoo on her breast in full bloom. She'd recovered well from her tuberculosis of a few years ago and then struggled with depression and crack cocaine use. She couldn't gain weight. Finally, with the help of her mother and sister, she got herself together and left the drugs behind. When the protease inhibitors came along she filled her prescriptions and took the pills. We had to change her medications a couple of times because one medication gave her terrible diarrhea and another made her hair fall out. Eventually she settled on a tolerable regimen that involved taking pills three times a day and she didn't miss a dose. Her viral load fell to an undetectable level and her CD4 cell count slowly rose.

"Hello, Dr. Ball," she said in her low, smoky voice. Her wavy black hair was pulled back in a loose ponytail and her full lips shone pink and wet.

"How are things going with you, Sophia?" She sat across from me in a purple halter top that revealed a bare midriff complete with pierced navel.

"I'm doing good." Her dark eyes sparkled and she smiled. "I'm taking all my medications and doing good."

"And you're still clean, right? No crack?"

"Oh, no. Not for a long time. Two years now, and never again," she said with a low laugh.

"That's great. Good for you. How is your weight?" I'd given her a medication to stimulate her appetite.

"Not so good." She looked down into the little black purse she carried and found a tissue. Her lip trembled. "I don't know, Dr. Ball. I have a good appetite and I eat good but I just can't gain no more weight. I can't get over a hundred and thirty-five pounds. I drink the Ensures from Miranda. I take the Megace that you give me." She dabbed at her eyes.

"Well, it might help if you stopped smoking."

"I know. I've cut down."

Patients always told me that they cut down. I guess it sounded better than saying "I'm smoking as much as I can," but I rarely considered "cutting down" to be anything close to quitting. Sophia had been through a lot, though, and I didn't want to push her on this. "I don't think that you should stress out about quitting smoking right now. Smoking's bad for you, it's bad for everyone. You'd probably gain some weight if you stopped, but I also think your sobriety, your staying clean, is really important. I'm not going to give you the hard sell today."

She blew her nose into the tissue and gave me a little smile.

"And how is the estrogen going? You're getting shots every two weeks or once a month now?"

"Every two weeks." When Sophia first came to me she'd been getting estrogen shots from the black market on the street. She had her own network of transgender friends who made their recommendations for which drugs would enhance the feminine look in a masculine body. Not having any training whatsoever in transgender medicine or pharmacology, I'd had to hunt down some articles to find out what doses would be safe and effective to prescribe for her. A well-known clinic downtown had a reputation as a center where transgendered individuals could get their care, and I'd consulted with the physicians there as well.

"Do you find that the estrogen affects your appetite at all?"

"No. The hormone shots don't make me hungry."

"I don't think the HIV meds are preventing you from gaining weight. Your counts are great: your last T cell count was up to four hundred and twenty-three. Your viral load is undetectable. I know you want to weigh more, but looking back, your weight has been pretty steady since you gained twenty pounds after the TB. It just may be that your body likes this weight and doesn't want to weigh more."

I took her blood pressure, looked at her throat, and listened to her heart and lungs. I felt her abdomen and wrote out the renewals for her medications. As she left I reassured her that she looked wonderful. She had appointments to see the nutritionist and the psychiatrist after me. I smiled to myself, remembering how sick she'd been a few years ago and how well she looked now. So many people hadn't made it to this point. We'd work on her smoking one of these days.

got back to my office after rounding on the inpatient floor to find Olive's chart waiting for me. She'd gotten the first appointment of the afternoon. Not surprisingly, the baby talk condition had never really amounted to anything. It didn't seem to bother Olive and we didn't leap to order tests or specialists. Olive's mother lived far away and the trauma of their visit together receded over the intervening weeks, as did the bizarre speech pattern that Olive had adopted in an apparent reaction to their meeting. Once in a while a random phrase or sentence would have an infantile quality to it. "It come and go," as Olive commented.

Olive always told us that she took her medication. Unfortunately, the test results didn't support this claim. If she was taking her medication, her viral load should be undetectable. According to her chart, the last labs had been done a month ago. Her viral load had risen to over fifty thousand copies after she'd initially had a good response. Olive took her pills faithfully for a few months and then seemed unable to maintain the adherence. It had happened several times already. She never admitted to not taking her medication but agreed to try something new when the current regimen seemed to be failing. I signed her up for a trial of a newer protease inhibitor that would be opening in a few weeks.

Despite the mantra "Hit early, hit hard," patients like Norbert and Olive forced us to realize that those who took their medication inconsistently could do themselves more harm than good. Patients who lacked understanding or commitment might never suppress their viral load and only create a virus that was increasingly resistant. We began to talk about the importance of adherence with our patients well before we even wrote a prescription for HIV treatment. The nurses at CSS did a great deal of teaching and the social workers, too, spoke to the patients about adherence.

Olive dragged herself across the waiting room when I called her name. She looked gloomy and sad, moving slowly. Her chart revealed that her weight had gone up four pounds since her last visit. Her hair today was done in dozens of tight yellow braids, with a small gold ornament affixed to the end of each strand. She came in and sat down.

"So how are things going?" I asked her.

"Not good. I'm still having that diarrhea. I go all day. I can't eat."

"This is the same diarrhea that you've been having right along? Nothing different?"

"The same." She sat in the chair a bit hunched over, looking uncomfortable.

"How many times have you gone to the bathroom so far today?"

"I didn't go yet today."

"Did you have breakfast today?"

"I had pancakes."

"And dinner last night, did you have dinner?"

"I had chicken and mashed potatoes last night."

"Well that sounds good. At least you're eating a bit, it seems." Didn't she just tell me that she couldn't eat? "We've done stool studies a few times for this diarrhea and so far the cultures have been negative. Do you take Imodium or Kaopectate?"

"Nothing works. I had some cheese sticks yesterday and I think that may have done it because I'm lactose intolerant." She gave a wan smile, saying, "I shouldn't eat anything with milk in it and I forgot that cheese is from milk."

I nodded, looking at her. "And how is the medication going?"

"Oh I'm taking it. I'm taking it because that's what's giving me all this diarrhea. I know it is. Every time I have to go to the bathroom."

"But you're not skipping doses at all?"

"No, you can ask my nurse. I take my meds."

I asked Olive to sit up on the examining table and I checked her blood pressure, heart, lungs, and abdomen. I found nothing abnormal. When I finished she sat down again in the chair in front of my desk and looked into her purse, pulling out a shiny white folder. "Here," she said, handing it over to me.

I saw bold red writing and recognized the outline of a cruise ship on the cover. I opened the folder to find an eight-by-ten glossy picture of Olive, with her yellow braids, wearing a long, draping purple gown and standing in front of a railing with an orange sunset behind her. She held a wineglass in her left hand.

"Wow," I said.

"Cancún," she said.

"Wow, that looks great, Olive. When were you there?"

"Two weeks ago. Mick and I went for a cruise." She looked very pleased.

I closed the folder and handed it back to her. "I'm totally jealous. Did you have a good time?"

"It was really nice. A very big ship, all new. It was their first cruise with that boat. The food was great." She took the folder and put it back into her purse.

"And was your diarrhea OK there?"

"Oh, I still had it on the cruise but I didn't let it bother me."

I nodded again. "Well, that's good. I'm glad that you had a good time. Thank you for showing me the picture." I'd been over territory like this before with Olive and each time it left me feeling off balance because her words and her actions were so out of sync. She couldn't eat but she ate pancakes and mashed potatoes and chicken and cheese sticks. She had diarrhea all day, every day, but had no difficulty going on a cruise. She complained and bent over in apparent discomfort and distress, yet there she was sipping wine on the deck, enjoying the sunset! I also felt annoyed at this incongruous presentation of hers and the role she seemed to want me to play: to admire her photo from Mexico but take seriously her reported symptoms and problems. She told me she took her HIV medications but her viral load reflected that she did not. Should I jump up and yell, "Liar, liar, pants on fire!"? The thought had definitely occurred to me.

"So, Olive, your viral load is up pretty high again and we're waiting for this study to open with the people down the hall." The AIDS Clinical Trials Group had its offices on part of the twenty-fourth floor with us. They did government- and pharmaceutical-sponsored studies of both approved drugs and those in development. Studies, for example, to see whether one regimen could be deemed superior to another, or whether certain regimens led to greater or lesser degrees of toxicity. Olive had already been screened to start on a regimen with a newer protease inhibitor in development. It would not be her first study. The coordinator and I had talked of Olive's adherence. As much as they wanted to get patients into the drug trials, a patient who didn't take the medication did not help their outcomes. We all hoped that this time her adherence would be better.

"Keep taking your medications as best you can, Olive. We'll keep an eye on the diarrhea for now. Let me know if it gets any worse. Hopefully the clinical trials people will be calling you soon."

As she left my office I wondered how long it would be before she really got sick.


After I'd seen my last patient of the afternoon, I went to rounds. Clinic had been busy and there were a lot of names to get through. Stan leaned back in his chair, the ever-present cup of coffee in his hand. Gerald read through the list name by name and the various providers who'd seen the patient that day gave their brief accounts. Brandon came late as usual, and when his patients' names were called, each time he said, "Doing fine, no problems today."

Occasionally he'd add some other detail if the patient had recently been in the hospital or started a new treatment regimen. He rarely looked up when the social worker or nurse talked about his patients. Although he continued to value the multidisciplinary approach at CSS, he often gave the impression that he found our clinic rounds a waste of time. No one appreciated Brandon's attitude less than Gerald, but the two ignored each other, which kept things calm.

I mentioned Norbert's new syphilis infection, voicing my concern over the dissemination of a resistant virus in the club scene.

"He's certainly not the only one," said Gerald, looking up from the sheets.

"I know," I agreed, "but I wish there was something more to offer than admonishment."

"You could call the cops," said Stan. He didn't mean it, of course. He felt just as powerless about this kind of thing as I did. We all protected our patients, acknowledging the stigma and prejudice that could be aimed at people with HIV. We believed fiercely in their autonomy, yet we could not always condone some of their behavior.

"I've talked to Norbert several times about safer sex," said Robert, an excellent nurse who'd started working with us last year. "He's certainly aware of the need for condoms but he has a lot of excuses for not using them. Even today, after getting his shots for syphilis, he told me that he thought condoms were for sissies."

"Oh great," I said, and several people around the table groaned.

"Well, there goes the neighborhood," said Stan, sipping his coffee and shaking his head.

"OK." Gerald looked down at the list and called Sabir's name.

"Sabir came in with his mother. I spoke to him alone for a bit and then his mother joined us. Sabir is looking pretty terrible, with KS over most of his face. He's been coming to CSS for about two years and at first wouldn't take HAART or accept any treatment for the KS. Then last year he did take meds for about nine months, during which time his lesions improved tremendously and he gained some weight. Unfortunately, his father died about four months ago. Even though they'd had a very conflicted relationship, Sabir seems to be mourning this loss by stopping all his meds."

I'd been so glad when Sabir had finally agreed to take HIV medication last year. His KS had responded beautifully to the improvement in his immune system. I tried to remember what, if anything, specifically led to Sabir's welcome change of attitude after all the months when I'd been frustrated and worried.

Then I recalled that Sabir had moved out of his own apartment and back into his parents' house. That had made the difference for him. When Sabir just recently told me that he didn't want to take medications anymore, he claimed that despite the improvement he'd experienced, he didn't want to live his life dependent on pills. In a conversation with Sabir's mother I'd subsequently learned of the father's death. With his father gone, Sabir's sad, self-destructive reaction was a return to his old stance against being on medications.

Paul Ferand had seen him today. "The mother is understandably very upset," he said. "At the same time, there seems to be some kind of shift in the hierarchical structure as Sabir is now the only male in that family. As much as he remains the youngest child, he is suddenly the patriarch and the mother is deferring to him and his decisions in a way that seems to be confusing for both of them. I spent a lot of time with them trying to get at the heart of this but I'm not sure they can see it. It's very enmeshed between mother and son, and the cultural influence is powerful as well. Meanwhile, Sabir's KS looks terrible. His T cells have plummeted. He's coming back to see you next week," he said, looking at me, "and I'll see him again then as well. I'll see him without the mother next time. I tried to offer him a low dose of an antidepressant but he isn't interested."

The room was quiet as we all listened to this dismaying story. Most of the people there knew of Sabir because the KS marked his face so prominently. Occasionally, when he sat in the waiting room, the whole place became more subdued. People avoided looking at him, and more than one patient had asked me about "the guy with the purple face" when they came into my office. Sabir. What could I say to him?

Gerald continued through the list of names. One of Stan's patients had told him, for the tenth time, that she was going to sue him. One of Dan's patients had eaten a ham sandwich throughout the visit. Briana couldn't get her patient to come out of the waiting room to talk to her, and Jeff couldn't get his patient out of his office so he could see other patients. Many patients were doing well on their medications. Others struggled with adherence or side effects, trying to find a regimen that they could tolerate. And then there were the patients telling their doctor that they took their medications when the labs revealed otherwise. Olive didn't have an exclusive hold on that phenomenon. Brandon had a patient who he thought was selling his prescriptions because he filled them right on time but his counts never budged. We knew of the increasing street value of the medications, and a couple of wily patients were cashing in, compromising their health to make money.

I told the group about Olive's glossy sunset portrait from the cruise ship in Mexico. Appreciative laughter greeted this report. Olive had her own notoriety at CSS for her years of various somatic complaints and her occasionally unique presentations. The baby talk episode had left quite an impression. I just wished she'd take her HAART so that her HIV would be under better control.

Finally the long rounds ended and most of the people in the room got up to leave. I sat there for a bit, letting the crowd file out, thinking about the busy day. Stan looked over at Brandon and said, "So. What happened?"

Brandon looked at him puzzled for a moment and then gave an embarrassed laugh. "How'd *you* find out?"

"Jean told me. The nurses all know."

"Well, word gets around fast," Brandon said.

"What?" I asked. I had no idea what they were talking about.

"His patient died at the airport," said Stan, looking at Brandon.

"*What?*" I definitely had not heard about this.

"You know, that patient—"

"Okindo," said Brandon.

"Okindo." Stan nodded. "The one we approved for the flight home."

"Oh yeah, that guy." I looked at Brandon. "Your patient who was dying and going back to Zambia . . ."

"Côte d'Ivoire," said Brandon.

"He died?"

Stan interjected, "So I get this call earlier—"

"They called you?" Brandon looked incredulous.

"Well, apparently the airline called the hospital; they had the clinic number but not your name. I got a call asking if I knew the patient. I gave them your name. They didn't say what was going on at the time."

Brandon shook his head. "We were just a few hours too late."

"So what happened?" Stan asked again.

"They called me and said, are you Dr. Barnes? Is this your patient? And I said yes. I'd written that detailed letter and cleared him to fly. I told them to read the letter. He was with the cousin who was taking him home. "

"When did you write the letter? Wasn't he supposed to go home last week?"

"Yeah, last week, it was set but then something with the cousin; he couldn't go until today."

"Sounds like it was a week late."

"Well, they said, Dr. Barnes, your patient is here in the departure lounge for the flight but he doesn't look very good. I said, I'm a physician. I've cleared the patient to fly. Yes, he's very sick. He's going home to be with his family. Next thing I know, not five minutes later they call to tell me he's dead."

"Oh my gosh, in the departure lounge?" I hadn't heard a thing about this all day. Totally out of the loop.

"Apparently he didn't even collapse or tip over; he was just sitting there. Dead." Brandon himself looked a bit stunned.

"So you're a physician? That's what you said to them?" Now Stan shook his head with a resigned smile. It sounded so ridiculous.

"I know, pretty fucking crazy, isn't it?" Brandon tried to smile back but the obscenity belied the sad truth of the matter. His patient hadn't made it home.

I'd once sent a patient home to Africa to die. A young woman with very young children and a bewildered husband. The woman had severe cerebral *Toxoplasmosis* and could not take several of the antibiotics that normally treated this condition. So she took second- and third-line drugs. There were many pills and she missed a lot of doses. She became more and more ill and we talked to her husband about her dying. They just wanted to go home to Mali. Dr. Jacobs gave the OK to use donated funds to buy her family their one-way tickets back. It was a horrible version of the American dream: to come to the United States from a third world nation, looking for a better life, find out you have AIDS, and then go back home to die. And yet we felt so lucky to be able to offer a ticket to the rare patient who needed it. Where else could they hope to receive a free trip home? I've always wondered what happened to my patient when she got off the plane. Did she see her mother or her sisters? Did she see the man who'd infected her before she set off to America with a new husband? And what happened to the children?

I had a macabre image of Brandon's dead patient sitting in the airport, waiting for his flight with all of the other passengers, while Brandon cavalierly told the dumbfounded airline attendants, "I'm a physician." I know he meant well; it took a lot of good intentions and hard work to organize such a trip for a dying patient. Despite myself, I was smiling too at the unpredictable way things had turned out, and the certain consternation of the poor cousin, the passengers, and the airline employees. A fellow passenger sitting there but already departed.

"Seems like he took a different flight." I commented sadly.

# Chapter Seventeen

# 1999 Coping with a Different Paradigm

My second son, Paris, born in 1998, would have been named Sarah, after my mother, but since he wasn't a girl, he was named after the city that she loved most. Jules had not known what to expect with the arrival of a sibling. He warily anticipated a being of similar size and temperament as himself. When we arrived at home after two nights away, Shari carried the tiny bundle in her arms. Paris slept quietly and Jules, taking a very relieved peek, said, "I will share all my toys with my new baby brother." We thought that was a very good start. My pregnancy had gone easily and the maternity leave passed before I could blink. Two small boys at home kept us constantly running. In addition, Shari's work as an obstetrician/gynecologist meant some very long nights and unpredictable hours. For me the patient flow at CSS never diminished. I had teaching and administrative responsibilities as well. At times I felt as if Sunday night came before last Monday even started.

Working with HIV-infected patients continued to offer a vibrant learning environment as well as unexpected situations. Armed with effective medicine to treat HIV, and having seen and heard the stories of near-miraculous recoveries in patients taking HAART, we'd unconsciously lulled ourselves into thinking that taking care of our patients could be straightforward, even easy. One by one, however, patients showed us how naïve this perspective could be.

It was five years since I'd first met Sabitha. By 1999 her four children were not so young any more, with the oldest daughter fifteen, the twins thirteen, and the "baby" eleven. We called them the feral children. Monica, the oldest, ran the show. Hardly ever in school, she gave the visiting nurses an impossible time, refusing to open the door, swearing at them, not following through on appointments. The twin boys cut classes and got into fights. The "baby," so far, had not had any mishaps. She did well in school and the nurses reported that she stayed out of trouble. The kids had lived with Sabitha's alcoholic mother during the months when she'd been in the nursing home. Once discharged, Sabitha happily moved back to her own apartment with her children, out from under her mother's roof.

The boyfriend stopped coming with her about six months after she left the nursing home. When I asked about him, Sabitha, smiling, shook her head. "He isn't comin' no more. Good riddance." Sabitha's Spanish-speaking home attendant listened quietly; she met my gaze and looked away. I wondered what had happened, but the boyfriend's absence didn't surprise me. I'd always been impressed by his devotion. He'd stuck with her, hung in there until she'd gotten home to her children. But I could see where a sustained relationship with Sabitha wouldn't work. She couldn't control her kids or her mother. No one could tolerate that situation for long. I missed his black baseball cap and the big faux diamond stud in his ear. More, I missed the stability and support that he'd provided for her.

Sabitha's home attendant spent eight hours a day at their apartment, helping Sabitha dress, cooking her meals, and accompanying her to the clinic. I'd heard firsthand stories of home attendants who could be unhelpful, dishonest, and lazy, but the woman who helped Sabitha was none of these. She stayed with Sabitha despite the wild children and the alcoholic mother. She went with her to the physical therapist and the neurologist and she wheeled Sabitha into my office every month or two. Sabitha's mother never came to CSS and I'd never seen her at the hospital. On rare occasions Monica came with her mother to an appointment. Home attendants were not allowed to dispense medications, but this quiet woman could at least report to me whether Sabitha was taking her pills or not. The home attendant proved to be the most steady, reliable person in Sabitha's world.

In the nursing home Sabitha's medications had been given to her and a nurse watched while she took them. This structured, regimented lifestyle saved her. The timing was fortunate: another few months and Sabitha likely would have been dead. Instead she started on a cocktail with protease inhibitors that halted the rapid deterioration and reversed some of the earlier neurological damage. In her first month at home Sabitha was seen every day by a visiting nurse who checked her blood pressure and general progress and oversaw the taking of the medications. After the first month these visits decreased to three times a week, and the chaos of Sabitha's family and her own lack of organization and commitment wrecked any consistent schedule. Within a few months her viral load started to go up. She'd give me a smile and shake her head. In her halting, nasal voice she'd say, "Those pills are too, too big," or "Sometimes I just forget," the words sticking to one another like Scotch tape. Her smile illuminated her face but no longer lit up the room, though she continued to look like a young girl, all ninety-five pounds of her sitting in the wheelchair.

When she'd first gone home Sabitha was able to get up with someone close by her, guiding her, and slowly walk using a walker. The physical therapist went to her home every day and expressed great optimism that she'd be walking well on her own in a matter of months. After a few weeks her insurance allowed for physical therapy only twice a week. She was given exercises to do each day. She never did them. When I asked if she walked at home with the walker she said yes and the home attendant shook her head. Sabitha smiled again as if the situation was funny. She said sometimes she used the walker to get herself to the bathroom. "I don't do the exercises. I guess I'm just lazy."

Monica often refused to allow the physical therapist into the house. She complained that he came late. Or too early. Before long the physical therapist stopped trying to go there at all. Sabitha remained in her wheelchair. And she didn't seem to mind. The kids pushed her around, took her to the store and to the park. The family had no household phone, a crazy situation that much hard work on the part of the CSS social worker failed to remedy. Monica had her own phone and gave us her number but she rarely answered if we tried to call. The mother, too, had a telephone but refused to give us her number. We could never confirm an appointment or let Sabitha know that her transportation was on its way. We tried to communicate by contacting the visiting nurse but this proved ridiculously difficult as well. There were times when no one answered the buzzer when the nurse went to the apartment and Monica didn't answer her phone. The height of absurdity came when we were reduced to calling the daughter of the home attendant in order to set up transportation to an appointment or a test for Sabitha.

With her viral load rising, I tried changing medications to get her HIV back under control. Sabitha could never adhere to a regimen. One pill gave her a headache, another pill made her vomit. One pill gave her diarrhea and another had to be taken too many times a day. Her neurologic condition deteriorated, with increased muscle jerking, more speech difficulties, and inability to move her legs. Her skin took on a dry, grayish hue and she began to complain of persistent nausea. The home attendant never let Sabitha lie to me about how consistently she did or didn't take her medication. But it seemed that as Sabitha got sicker, her tolerance for the pills lessened. The medication became an enormous burden. Finally, at one visit I suggested she take a break for a few weeks and not take anything at all. Both of them looked relieved that I hadn't tried to get her to take yet another impossible pile of medications.

That night Stan telephoned.

"Sorry to call you at home. Your patient's mother called the clinic after hours and threatened to come after you and stab you."

"What? Who?" I stood in my kitchen making salad dressing for our dinner. The boys were asleep.

"Sabitha L. Her mother called the service and was very loud and angry. They called me and I called her back."

"What did she say?"

"That you didn't give her daughter any medication and she's very sick and the mother is going to stab you."

I started to laugh at how crazy it sounded. "The patient didn't want to be on medicine, the mother has never once shown her face or called me, and now this? Is there something I should do?"

"I called security, just to be sure. They have some kind of protocol for this type of thing and they take it seriously. They told me to call you and make you aware of the threat."

"MD aware." This was a deadpan phrase we used when nurses or administrators gave us information only for the sake of letting us know: information that required no intervention or order on our part but would, by our knowing, shift the responsibility to us. "The patient in room twenty-six had a bowel movement." "MD aware." That kind of thing.

"Well," I continued, "I'm glad you told me. The mother is really a bad alcoholic, according to Sabitha. I've never met her but apparently she is pretty out there. And I seem to recall that she's been in jail for stabbing someone." I remembered Sabitha telling me this one day; it seemed a very long time ago.

"Oh great. Hopefully she's doing more drinking than stabbing these days," Stan said.

"So do I do anything different?" I wondered if there was a protocol for my response.

"I think they just want you to be aware of it, aware of your surroundings, especially at the hospital. Security will have someone wander through the clinic a couple of times tomorrow. Other than that I don't think there's anything special. Sorry to call you at home. It's suspiciously quiet there." I could hear a young child fussing in the background on his end of the phone line.

"Yeah, they're both asleep for the moment. Paris will be up in an hour or two. Is that Charlie I hear?"

"No, it's Lizzie. An earache." He groaned. Stan's household had too much experience with earaches.

"I'm sorry you got bothered with this. Thanks for letting me know. I'll be on the lookout tomorrow for a crazy drunken woman with a knife in her hand." I didn't actually feel as jaunty as I might have sounded. No one had ever threatened me before. That it came from someone I'd never even seen made it all the more bizarre and unnerving. I got off the phone just as Shari came into the kitchen and I told her the story.

She shook her head, saying, "You sure do have some wild stories, Dr. Balls. Let's make sure the door is locked."

We checked the door and then had dinner.


Nothing came of Sabitha's mother's threat. I was a little more tense than usual at work for a couple of days, always looking up and down the hall when I left my office. But we never heard another word about it, and when I next saw Sabitha I didn't mention it to her.

Funnily enough, however, a few weeks later one of the patients came to clinic with the handle of a very large knife poking out of the back of his pants. He paced around near the elevators while Stan and one of the nurses went out and quietly escorted the other patients from the waiting room down to the conference room. We waited for security to come.

I was with a patient, Loretta. "That guy is on a mission," she told me.

"What does that mean?" I asked.

"A mission. You know, a mission. He needs some crack. He's on a mission." Loretta had been my patient for a few years, a small, dark-haired woman with dark eyes circled with kohl and the parched voice of too many cigarettes. She sat across from me in my office with a knowing look.

"Really?" I hadn't heard this expression before. I had only just glimpsed the guy out in the waiting room, having been warned, along with the other staff, of this unexpected menace. He looked disheveled, his khaki pants baggy, yellow shirt untucked, long, dark wavy hair in need of a wash.

"I know. That guy is on a mission. I recognize it. Any crackhead would. I seen it many times." Loretta had been there. She'd first come to me after spending a year in a halfway house getting off drugs. She'd been clean ever since, a feat I increasingly appreciated, as crack had a very alluring hold on people even after many months without it.

"He's on a mission for crack? Why would he come here?"

"Doesn't he have an appointment?" Loretta looked surprised.

I burst out laughing. "Well, nobody's got any crack here!"

She smiled, raising her eyebrows. "Maybe he knows another patient here."

I hadn't thought of that. I wished he hadn't brought that enormous knife on his mission. "Goodness, I hope the security guards get him before he decides to take his knife out of his pants."

"Oh, he probably won't hurt anybody. He just wants his crack."

Later in rounds Stan referred to the patient as "Machete Man." The security guards had come up the back stairs and with Stan, Gerald, and Dr. Ferand they went out to the waiting room where the patient was quietly pacing. Stan's size helped; Machete Man barely came up to his shoulder. We all secretly suspected that the security guards were happy to have Stan with them as well. Without any yelling or drama, he gently told the guy that we couldn't have him in the clinic with a knife. He didn't object, peacefully handing it over, and he quietly got onto the elevator with the guards. Stan gave a very big sigh of relief when that episode was over. In rounds Gerald thanked us all for our calm and commented on how the patients had been fairly unfazed by the whole thing. I relayed Loretta's pronouncement that he'd been on a mission. Other people in the room nodded, having heard the term before. Stan observed that this sort of mission would not be under Sister Harriet's purview.

"Do you think we need to kick him out?" Gerald asked.

"Uh, yeah," said Stan emphatically. "I don't want to be taking machetes away from crackheads up here any more than I have to."

The patient had never been known as a troublemaker or a difficult guy, but we all felt that bringing a weapon to clinic provided more than adequate grounds for discharging a person from our care. Gerald would write him a letter and we'd make sure that he had a thirty-day supply of medication and a list of other HIV clinics in the city. Machete Man would not be the first patient to receive such a letter. Nor, of course, the last.

In the summer of 1999 I experienced my first day in seven years without an inpatient to visit in the hospital. My office hours were very busy, as my outpatient panel had nearly doubled. But that one day came as an explicit reminder of how far we had come in our ability to treat HIV and AIDS. From those first cases in 1981, the death rates from AIDS had steadily risen until a certain point in the early 1990s when AIDS became the leading cause of death among people aged twenty-five to forty-four. In 1995, at the height of the epidemic in the United States, nearly fifty thousand people died of AIDS in one year and the numbers continued to rise. But the protease inhibitors changed everything. By 1999 the annual number of deaths from AIDS had fallen to fewer than eighteen thousand.

This dramatic decrease in deaths meant that fewer people needed hospitalization. Obviously no one objected to this remarkable success, but the hospital didn't make money if it didn't have patients in the beds. So we needed more patients. In order to care for those patients with HIV who required hospitalization, we needed to see a lot more outpatients. Our panels grew and we hired another doctor and more staff. Our fifth doctor came from a research position at the Rockefeller Institute. He was a quiet, extremely caring and likeable fellow named Aaron. His panel started from zero. With referrals from all over the city, including the prison system (better known by some as "the island"), other HIV clinics, word of mouth, and new patients in the hospital, Aaron quickly built a busy panel. One of his patients was a very flamboyant transgendered woman who adored him. She'd sashay down the hall to his office, jiggling her many bracelets and swinging her hips. He'd smile and calmly hold the door for her, never giving her less than his full respect and attention. Though a "new doc" at our site, he proved a welcome addition and very soon hit his stride among all the demands and the crazy characters, both patients and providers.

Dr. Jacobs, Stan, and Gerald put together a huge proposal to open up a satellite clinic at the site of the new Gay Men's Health Crisis building downtown. Any patients seen in the downtown clinic who needed to be hospitalized would come uptown for that purpose. The proposal was accepted by GMHC and our hospital. In preparation for this undertaking we hired five more doctors and all the attendant support staff needed for our multidisciplinary approach, including psychiatrists, nurses, social workers, nutritionists, lab technicians, secretaries, and administrators.

The intense intimacy of working at CSS changed. It didn't happen in one day or one month, but as we expanded to accrue more patients, and as the downtown site got up and running, more and more new people sat in on clinic rounds and support group and on Fridays for inpatient conference. Our patients were no longer dying in the harrowing numbers of just a few years ago. The very real need for support and togetherness with my colleagues gradually evolved into a less close-knit, less consuming connection. The new physicians came from training in infectious diseases, and the social workers almost always seemed young. The nursing staff increased and we hired a new nutritionist. I had more autonomy at work. We all did. We simply didn't know one another as well as we used to, and we didn't know one another's patients quite as well either. It took some time for me to appreciate this change in the environment at CSS.

My single day of not rounding in the hospital did not occur again for quite a while. There were always patients needing hospitalization, though it might not be for an HIV-related cause. And although some days I spent less time rounding, I made up for it in office hours, teaching the medical students, supervising the residents, running a lecture series, serving on hospital committees, writing articles, and doing paperwork.

One day as I sat at my desk going through charts and calling patients, the front desk buzzed me on the intercom to say that a doctor with an unpronounceable name was calling from an outside hospital in another part of the city. I took the call.

"This is Dr. Ball."

"Hello, my name is Dr. Srinivastenandu. I'm an infectious diseases attending at Mercy Overbridge. How are you?" Whoever she was, she had a lovely voice with a pronounced Indian accent.

"I'm fine," I said. "What can I do for you?"

"I'm calling about a patient whom I believe you may know. Her name is Peaches M."

"Oh yes, I know Peaches. Is she there at your hospital?" Immediately I thought of Peaches yelling "I'M DYIN'!" into the phone. I hadn't seen her in over a year.

"I'm afraid that she's passed away. She died yesterday here on our medical floor."

I looked around my office. Everything seemed the same. There was my examining table with the white paper pulled to the end. The "on" switch of the otoscope glowed green and I realized I should have turned it off. My sweater hung neatly on a hanger on the back of my door. The light from the window behind me came into the room as it always had, highlighting the dust between the keys on my computer keyboard, falling on the colorful tempera paintings that Jules had done in nursery school which I'd taped to the wall on my right. Just the other day Ernie, an extremely lovable character, a patient, had asked me if I thought Jules would grow up to be an artist. Ernie had twin boys he adored but he got mixed up with crack, lost his marriage, and didn't get to see his boys very often. He told me some hair-raising stories about trying to haul himself away from drug use and back to his sons. Once he came in with a black eye the size of a grapefruit after he'd confronted four drunk twenty-year-olds and their baseball bat. He'd gotten angry at them when they shouted at his dog.

"Hello?"

Right. It was that doctor from Overbridge, the one with the very long name.

"Yes." I said. "Yes, I'm sorry. I just wasn't expecting this. Can you tell me what happened?"

"Well, she was admitted here four days ago. She came in with abdominal pain and fever. We believe that she had a perforated bowel from a mycobacterial abscess."

"Oh, I'm so sorry to hear this news."

"I'm sorry to be the one to tell you. I saw from the chart that the patient wanted us to call you when she first came in by ambulance, but she deteriorated very quickly here and I think they were focused on her medical problems. No one seems to have seen those notes. She couldn't really speak after that. I take it her HIV was not under control?"

"No, not at all. She had a very hard time taking her medication. She'd never had an opportunistic infection but her T cells were low and she had a lot of skin rashes."

"Yes, we could tell. Her CD4 cell count here was only two."

"I'm not surprised. It wasn't TB, was it?"

"No, it looks like *Mycobacterium avium*. And also some pseudomonas grew in her blood."

"Oh boy." I sighed. "Her children are quite young."

"Yes, I know. Our social workers have been in touch with an uncle somewhere in the city. It's not clear what is going to happen with the boys. We couldn't locate the father."

"I think there are several fathers."

"Ah. That could make it complicated. We hope that the uncle will help us."

"I appreciate your calling to let me know. We were very fond of Peaches here. She was quite a personality."

"Well, thank you for taking my call."

I hung up and gazed around my office again. How could everything look the same? Out there somewhere were four boys whose lives were now utterly changed. I knew them only from their wild, exuberant screaming on the other end of the phone line. I pictured them laughing a lot, as Peaches had done, but tenderhearted, too, and honest about their feelings. The boys deserved a better chance. I closed my eyes and wished them well, hoping they'd remember Peaches's love and not her bad decisions or her drug use. I wished I'd been able to get her to take her medication. Her death gave me an empty feeling and, looking at my hands resting on the computer keyboard, I wondered what more I could have done. I couldn't make Peaches be someone she was not.

After two years without any word, Etta's name showed up on my schedule in the late fall of 1999. She had dropped completely out of sight and I didn't even know the outcome of her pregnancy. I hadn't expected her to write us postcards, but seeing her name suddenly brought up a lot of questions: Had her pregnancy been healthy? If there was a baby, was the baby HIV-negative? Would Etta still be on her medications? And where had she been?

She'd lost weight. From across the waiting room I could see that her face was a pasty color and her cheekbones stood out. As she came toward me I saw the cracked lips beneath the pink lipstick and the crooked application of eyeliner. Her jeans and her navy winter coat both seemed too large.

I held the waiting room door open for her. "You look like you don't feel very well," I said as she walked with me to my office.

"One of my eyes is blurry." She walked slowly and didn't look at me as she spoke.

"Come in and sit down. I'm happy you're here. It's been nearly two years. What's going on with you?"

"I wanted to come back. They don't know what they're doing at that other place."

"So you've been in care? Were you still going to the same place in Queens?"

"Not really. I mean sometimes. They got on my nerves." As she sneered in a familiar way a glimmer of her feistiness shimmered beneath the pallor.

"When was the last time you saw anyone there?"

She stared up at the ceiling for nearly ten seconds. I almost looked up there myself as she took so long to answer the question. "May," she finally said. "I think I went there in May."

"Did they have you on medication?"

"Oh, please." She waved her hand in disgust. "Every time I went there they gave me more pills. After a while it gets ridiculous, you know? But the last straw was the eye doctor there who wanted to put a needle in my eye. For what? I asked him, and he said it was an infection from childhood. Cider mug virus or something like that." She shook her head disparagingly and crossed her arms. "Uh-uh. No needles in my eye."

"That was in May?" CMV retinitis. Etta's in trouble. "And have you been taking the medications they gave you?"

"Like I said, it got ridiculous. But I probably need something at this point. I was sick of those people, though, so I came back to you."

"OK, great," I said, looking at her and taking a deep breath. "You said your eye is blurry now. You look like you've lost some weight as well."

"Yeah." She started picking at the remaining chip of red polish on her thumbnail. With a growing sense of apprehension I noticed the dry, brittle hair and the dry skin.

"Etta, the last time I saw you, you were pregnant. How did that go?"

"Oh fine. She's fine. She's at my mother's now, though, for this week. I needed to sleep."

"And she's negative?"

"Yeah. They gave her AZT. Which I wasn't too happy about, but, whatever."

"Well, congratulations, that's great. So you had the baby and were you fine too, then?"

"Yeah. For a while I was fine." She stopped picking at her nail. "But I don't know, with the baby and Joey I wasn't taking the medication right so they switched me to some other stuff but it made me totally sick so then they tried something else. I took it for a while. Some huge pills, then they wanted me to take even more pills. Ugh." She waved her hand again.

"How long have you been losing weight?"

"I don't know. I was one ninety when I had the baby. Then I was down to one seventy for a while."

"Do you remember how much you weighed at your appointment in May?" I saw on today's cover sheet that the nurses had recorded her weight as 123 pounds.

"I think I was about one sixty then. In the summer my appetite got bad."

"What else? Have you had any fevers? Coughing? Is your breathing OK?" She said no to each of these last questions. She complained of night sweats and a general sense of fatigue. When I examined her, what she called blurriness turned out to be nearly complete blindness in the bad eye. She hadn't realized how much her vision had deteriorated. I looked at the back of her eyes with the ophthalmoscope and saw some white patches. She'd need a thorough eye exam by the ophthalmologist, but on the basis of her story I felt certain she had cytomegalovirus. I also noted thrush on the sides of her mouth and a rapid heart rate.

"Etta, do you know what your last T cell count was?"

"Not good. I think it was like twelve or something."

As I washed my hands after examining her, I tried to organize my thoughts. Etta's exam heightened my concern. Between the weight loss and the low T cells, Etta's situation gave me a sinking feeling. Cytomegalovirus is an infection of very advanced AIDS. I turned back to talk to her; she sat on the table, looking too thin and sick. "Etta, the 'cider mug virus' that the eye doctor was telling you about is something called cytomegalovirus, or CMV. It's an infection that most of us get when we're kids and our immune systems fight it off so it never causes any problems. In people who have severe weakness of their immune systems, as in AIDS patients, or in some people who get transplants, the CMV comes back. In HIV patients it comes back most frequently in the eye and can make people blind. That's what's happening to that eye now. I want you to see the eye doctor here to be sure. You have some thrush, that's easy enough to treat, but this big weight loss is also worrisome. You haven't been here in a while and I don't want you to go home and not come back. You need to be in the hospital. Right now. Your eye needs to be treated today if not six months ago."

She'd gone back to picking at her nail polish as I spoke. She hadn't flinched when I said the word "blind." In the silence after my spiel I could hear one of the social workers laughing out in the hall. Etta looked up. "I kind of knew that you'd say that. About needing to be in the hospital."

Two years ago her willingness to cooperate would have been very unusual. She'd been going blind at home with two small children and now she could no longer handle it alone.

"I'm sorry. I'm sorry to see you looking so tired."

"Yeah, well." She put her head back and stared at the ceiling again for a moment. "I'm not happy about it either."

I had her lie down in the room next door while I made the five or six phone calls necessary to arrange for the ophthalmologist to see her, for her to get admitted, to talk to the admitting resident and the intern and tell the nurses to draw her blood and arrange transport for her. By some great piece of luck, there was a bed in the hospital that she could go to directly, without spending hours or the entire night in the emergency room.

Molly, Etta's social worker, went in to talk to her about staying in the hospital, making sure that the kids were taken care of. Etta called her grandfather to check that Joey would be picked up after school. Afterwards, Molly told me that Etta had talked about Joey having a hard time at home. Between the baby and Etta becoming more and more run down, he'd certainly felt overwhelmed, but as a young boy he wasn't well equipped to handle his feelings. He misbehaved a lot, throwing things and yelling, saying that he didn't like his baby sister, getting in trouble in school. One day Etta had found Joey squeezing himself onto the shelf under the kitchen sink. "He knows something's up with Etta," Molly said. "He told her he wanted to get into the refrigerator but he was too big. He doesn't have the maturity to articulate what he feels and Etta doesn't have the insight. It's sad. Wanting to get into the refrigerator, that kid's trying to figure out how to preserve himself," she said, leaving the office.

I went back into the room where Etta rested with her eyes closed. I couldn't help thinking about how well she'd done for that brief period before and during her pregnancy. Maybe that had been her plan all along, to take her medications and get her counts up so that she could have a healthy baby. Or maybe it just happened that way; she did well, she felt better, she went back to her usual stomping grounds and hooked up with the guy who bought her drinks. Well, now she had a little girl at home as well as a little boy.

I thought of my two little boys. Jules built fantastic cars and spaceships out of boxes and couch pillows. Eighteen months old, Paris woke up smiling every morning and blew a soft raspberry on my cheek with a low chortle when I held him in my arms. They needed me. And I needed them. Perhaps Etta's connection with her children came from basic but ephemeral instinct. She'd take care of them for a while, but how long? At this rate, how long? Then she'd be gone. They would live on without her.

"Etta," I said quietly. Slowly, she opened her eyes.

"Etta, you know, I didn't ask you before. What's your baby's name?"

"I named her Etta."

# Chapter Eighteen

# 2000 Going Home

We sat around the big table, Janice listening attentively as one of the new social workers, Gary, raised the issue that it was hard to be in a support group where the boss was also in the room. Gary said he didn't feel at ease stating what was on his mind. That was the day I realized that support group had ended. It had been coming for a while. At first so many new people meant that nearly all the chairs in the room were taken. But as we steadily got bigger over the last two years, what had once been an intimate, encouraging environment where we talked freely about the pain of caring for dying patients had instead become a place of guarded self-expression and scattered complaints about a difficult interaction with the Medicaid office or the frustration of a nursing home application.

I found myself going to support group less and less often, struggling with a guilty feeling as Janice, who still ran the sessions, had become my friend and I didn't want to disappoint her. She puzzled over the direction of the group, but after a while it became clear that the changes at CSS reflected the changes in the care and treatment of HIV and AIDS. We had more and more patients coming to our clinic, and in response our staff had grown in size as well. Patients continued to get sick, and some of them died. Still, there had been a distinct shift. The terrible days of no treatment, no options, and little hope became a part of our lore, not a part of our current reality.

The need for mutual support and comfort in times of intense emotional stress and anxiety had made support group a vital aspect of my early years at CSS. All of us benefited from those twice-monthly sessions when we were feeling helpless and our patients died. But by late 1999 I didn't need it as badly. And we'd gotten so big; around the table I saw too many unfamiliar faces to feel comfortable expressing my fears or my sadness. The shared history of those dark days before HAART wasn't something the new people could ever really understand. The multidisciplinary approach to patient care still guided our management but we couldn't all know one another as intimately as we once had. Dr. Jacobs had never been one to talk a lot in support group but he'd always been there as a presence, a quiet witness to his team's work and struggles. To a new young social worker Dr. Jacobs's natural shyness may have made him seem remote. Gary's words reflected the greater distance that now separated the boss and the social worker. Despite her great skills as our group's facilitator, Janice couldn't change that.

I looked across the table to where Dr. Jacobs sat, as usual, in a chair against the wall, gazing at the floor. I felt annoyed at the naïve social worker. Dr. Jacobs created something remarkable when he founded the Center for Special Studies. My admiration for him had only grown over the years as he remained steadfastly committed to the Center's providing "one-class care" to our patients. At a medical institution and teaching hospital as huge as ours there could be a lot of pressure to treat the rich patients differently from the poor. Our patients were not wealthy or famous or powerful. They weren't television personalities and they didn't come with bodyguards. Still, Dr. Jacobs made all of our jobs easier by having us approach our work with one simple rule: Do what is best for the patient. Support group had helped us all over the years to stay focused on that goal. Our support group, with its multidisciplinary attendees, had kept most of us from despair in those dark, dark days of the early 1990s. Dr. Jacobs benefited along with the rest of us. The social worker objecting to Dr. Jacobs's presence missed the point. But he was coming late to the party; in fact we didn't need the support group as much anymore.

And yet, though our need for support group might have diminished, our patients still needed us, some of them desperately.

On a Tuesday, shortly after she'd gotten back from a trip to Spain, Olive called to say she'd been having fevers for four days and a dry, painful cough. Although I was tempted to suggest she go to the emergency room, I asked her to come in to see me in the clinic. By early afternoon she was sitting in the waiting room coughing and looking tired. I brought her down to the lab to check the oxygen saturation in her blood with a little gadget I placed on her finger. After the brief walk down the hall she was breathing rapidly and her saturation measurement was low. She had a fever as well. We went back to my office.

"When did your fevers start?" I asked her as I sat down at my desk.

"Four days ago." She stopped to take a couple of breaths. "We got back a week ago Saturday and on Friday night I had a fever."

"And the cough?"

"I started coughing a little on the trip. I didn't pay it any attention." She stopped again. "I thought it was my asthma, that I was allergic to something."

"And this shortness of breath, did that start with the cough?"

"Worse over the weekend." Breath. "I didn't really notice it but maybe it started on the trip, too."

I pulled up her laboratory data on my computer and saw that her most recent CD4 cell count was six, not enough T cells to fight off much of anything. She didn't take Bactrim, either, as she had a sulfa allergy. The second choice for prophylaxis against *Pneumocystis* pneumonia did not work nearly as well. "I think we need to worry about PCP," I told her. "Your T cells are so low that you could have any number of infections in your lungs, but the most likely thing by far is *Pneumocystis*."

She nodded, closing her eyes. I looked at her and yet again felt tempted to address the topic of her poor adherence. The drug trial we'd been waiting for had been delayed several times and Olive remained on a regimen that didn't control the virus. I wrote the prescriptions and she claimed that she took her medications, but her viral load told a different story. With every new regimen she'd do well for a while, even getting her viral load down to undetectable levels. But each time, after a few months, the levels would rise again. She'd bat her eyelashes and look very surprised, saying, "I don't know why my viral load is up again." But she didn't try very hard to convince me and she never took offense when I pointed out the inconsistency between her lab results and what she was telling me. I never said to her, or to any patient, "You're lying." Sometimes I wanted to. I tried hard to accept that a patient might find it necessary to swear adherence even when we both knew it couldn't be true. I could only try my best to get my patients onto medications that worked and that they could tolerate. I stressed the importance of taking the medication correctly, but once a patient left my office I couldn't control what happened.

Taking medication seems straightforward and easy. It also seems that you could predict that a homeless or drug-using patient would take his or her medication much less regularly than a patient with a more stable environment. But studies from fifty years ago of patients on tuberculosis medications demonstrated that, on the contrary, it's impossible to predict which patients will or won't take their medication as prescribed. The rich banker might skip her pills just as often as the drug addict, and a homeless man could be meticulously attentive, never skipping a single dose. Still, treatment regimens for HIV in 1999 meant several pills, several times a day, not always an easy task for patients who didn't get breakfast every morning or might not brush their teeth every day. The troubles with adherence, one of the crucial aspects of caring for patients with HIV, began to emerge as emblematic of the deeper, more entrenched difficulties that plagued so many of my patients' lives. That taking medication proved so problematic exposed a reality of our society that had been somewhat obscured in those despairing times of relentless illness and no treatment. One by one, patients like Olive and Peaches, Sabitha and Norbert showed us that AIDS was just one piece of a life clouded by lacks or misfortunes of some kind. Poverty, abuse, absent parents, drugs, violence, mental illness, poor education: all these things and more provided the permanent background for so many of my patients and their families. AIDS on top of this became just another surge of water in an unrelenting storm.

I called the resident to arrange for Olive to be admitted and spoke to the intern who would be assigned to the case.

"Hi, Terry, it's Susan Ball at CSS. I'm admitting a patient of mine from clinic. I just wanted to let you know about her."

"Hi, Dr. Ball."

Terry Rosner had taken care of previous patients of mine and I found her direct, warm, and smart. Olive would be in good hands and I related the story briefly. "She'll need an ABG when she gets to you," I said. "I don't think she needs the intensive care unit but I could be wrong about that." ABG stood for arterial blood gas; it gave us information regarding how well the patient's lungs exchanged oxygen and carbon dioxide.

"OK, we'll do that first thing once she gets over here."

"You've taken care of patients with PCP before, haven't you?"

"Yes. Last month one of Dr. M.'s patients was here with PCP, and when I did the MICU last summer there were a couple of patients."

The protease inhibitors and the effectiveness of PCP prophylaxis had contributed to a significant drop in hospital admissions for this illness. I hadn't admitted a patient with PCP in more than six months. Five years ago I would have had two or three patients with *Pneumocystis* in the hospital at any given moment. In those days the residents admitted a patient with PCP at least once a week, often directly to the medical intensive care unit, with imminent respiratory failure. Usually these were patients with previously unknown HIV, or perhaps someone who knew his or her diagnosis but hadn't gone to the doctor. Now, with such a decline in cases, a resident might spend the whole rotation in the ICU without seeing a single case of PCP.

"Well," I said, "just as a reminder, they can get worse before they get better. It's not certain that she has PCP but it's definitely highest on the list of possibilities. Pulmonary should see her as well."

"OK. We'll call them. Dr. Ball, her T cells are so low. Shouldn't they be better on those medicines she's on?"

"Adherence has really been an issue for her. I've left her on this regimen but I'm not sure how much she takes or even if she takes it at all. She's scheduled to start on a study with one of the newer protease inhibitors but the study isn't open yet. I don't know if this infection will delay things or not."

"Should we keep her on her meds while she's here?"

"Hmmm. That's a good question." If we ordered the medication she'd get it in the hospital, whereas at home she apparently wasn't taking her pills. It would be like starting a new regimen for her. I wasn't sure that would be the right thing to do. "I don't think she's been taking anything in recent weeks. Let's keep her off for right now, until she's more stable."

"Sounds good. We'll keep a close eye on her. If the ABG is bad we'll get the MICU involved."

"Thanks." I gave her my beeper number and told her to page me if there were any questions.

A few minutes later my phone rang again.

"Hi, Dr. Ball, it's Terry again. I'm sorry to call you back but I wanted to check in with you about your other patient, Ms. B."

"Oh, of course, sorry." In my concern for getting Olive's admission settled I'd forgotten that Terry also took care of Etta. "I'm glad one of us can keep a thought in her head."

"Oh, I know how it is, believe me," she said. "I meant to call you earlier. She's not looking good. I saw your DNR order from late yesterday. Ophtho left a note that they want to do her implant tomorrow. She's still having fevers and we've had to lower her dose of ganciclovir because of her anemia."

"Yes, I know, I saw the notes." I looked out at the gray December skyline. I could see the wake of a boat moving up the East River. In the far distance the lights of the cars on the Major Deegan blinked white and red. I sighed. This was Etta's third week in the hospital. With a steady, sad progression the cyto-megalovirus had indeed infected her eye but hadn't stopped there. She had virus in her blood and we assumed the lesions in her brain came from it as well. In addition, she'd developed heart failure and although we didn't have a biopsy to prove it, we strongly suspected that the muscles of her heart were also infected with CMV. Her T cell count upon admission registered two. The medication for CMV caused suppression of the bone marrow, which resulted in her becoming severely anemic. Etta's HIV demonstrated resistance to all the medications that we could offer her. She'd looked bad when I admitted her just three weeks ago but now we were being squeezed into a very tight corner. I recognized the bitter familiarity of no options.

Last night I had spoken with Etta and her mother about what would happen if Etta stopped breathing. Mostly it was just Mrs. B. and me talking. Though awake, Etta could not focus on the decision whether she wanted to be on a breathing machine or not, should the need arise. With Etta deteriorating daily and our treatment options shrinking to zero, Etta's mother agreed that the do not resuscitate order should be placed in her chart.

To Terry I said, "That MRI of her brain definitely looks ominous. I had a good talk with the mother last night and she'll be in again this afternoon."

She paused for a moment before asking, "Is there anything else you'd like us to do? Should I tell ophtho to schedule her?"

"No, I don't think so. She doesn't seem to be in any pain and if anything these brain lesions have made her a bit out of it so I don't think she's suffering. It's nice that ophtho wants to do the procedure but I don't think it's going to make any difference."

I had tracked down the attending at the hospital in Queens from her admission there last May. He remembered Etta, noting that she'd been stubborn about refusing care for her eye. Despite their efforts to get her on an effective anti-HIV regimen, she'd been unwilling or unable to follow their suggestions. Now it was months later, and for most of those months Etta had been entirely out of care. In the last three weeks we'd slowed the process at best, but I knew of no new medications that would suddenly rescue her, as the protease inhibitors had done just a few years ago.

"Terry, I think you guys are doing what you can. Let's keep her on that lower dose of ganciclovir and watch her blood pressure. I'll be by this afternoon to talk to her mom when she's here."

"OK, Dr. Ball. We'll talk to ophtho. Let me know if you want anything else for her. We asked the nurses if she could be moved into a private room."

"Thanks." A private room would be nice for Etta. Maybe we could sneak the kids in for a visit. Technically they were too young to be visitors in the hospital, but the nurses could bend the rules at times.

In these three weeks I had gotten to know Etta's mother, a strong-willed, practical woman who lived in New Jersey, where she worked as a bookkeeper. Etta had chosen to live in the apartment building in Queens near her grandparents when Joey was born. Mother and daughter had a fractious relationship and the grandparents provided child care and many meals for Etta, especially in the periods when she was ill. With the birth of Etta's daughter nearly two years ago, Mrs. B. had come back into Etta's life, taking care of the children on the weekends and visiting more frequently. Etta's stubbornness and independence had originally driven her and her mother apart, but they seemed to have gotten over it. With Etta now in the hospital her mother came nearly every afternoon, after work, to see her daughter. I spoke to her a few times a week either in person or on the phone. Mrs. B. asked good questions and struggled to put up with the many small hassles of caring for someone in the hospital. Etta's room changed and no one let the mother know. Etta was scheduled for a test and had to miss a meal but then the test was canceled and no one remembered to order a tray. These things infuriated Etta's mother, but she was never unreasonable or overbearing with me. I'd learned a lot about Etta from her mother. The two of us had been able to laugh together over our frustration at how hard-headed Etta could often be. I recognized that Etta's personality was not terribly dissimilar from her mother's. Mrs. B. saw this as well.

Sometimes when I met with her at Etta's bedside I found it difficult to control my emotions. Etta's children were so young and it always reminded me of my own two little boys. I had to force myself not to imagine what it would be like for my sons to lose me. And my own mother's death still caught me at times. I found myself missing her with a catch in my throat. Yet here was a woman with a dying daughter. Mothers should not experience the death of their child. AIDS killed so many parents and children. The whole thing felt wrong. We had good medicine. Why did it have to be like this?

After I hung up the phone with Terry, I went out to the waiting room to call in my next patient. It struck me with a pang how normal Roman looked as he got up and walked toward me. He wore a stylish tan overcoat and dark green corduroy slacks. His tortoiseshell glasses made him look like an English professor, an appearance accentuated by the long hair brushed back from his face. You would never guess that those blue eyes crinkling in a smile had once been nearly covered with the purple lesions of Kaposi's. Roman's health had never taken a downward turn once he got on his HAART. In four years he could count on one hand the number of doses of medications he'd missed. Three times a day, every day. His viral load remained undetectable, and his T cells had risen slowly and steadily from the single digits to the hundreds, two hundreds, three hundreds. His, thankfully, was not the only success story in my practice, but it always made me happy to see him. I found it almost hard to imagine now that he'd been covered with KS, with a chest X-ray that revealed lungs full of lesions. Had he not started taking an effective regimen when he did, I had no doubt he'd have been dead within months, maybe weeks. And instead here he was looking fit and relaxed in a chair in my office.

"Roman, you look great."

"I'm feeling fine. Will you be checking my blood today?"

"Your last labs were done in July when you were here. The time passes quickly. It looks like you missed an appointment in October, so, yes, we'll do your labs today. Do you have enough medication?"

He nodded yes. "I called for refills last month."

"And you're still just as steady with taking your pills?"

He nodded again. "I never miss them. Why would I miss them now? They are no trouble." His accent created an almost musical quality to his voice.

"I'm so glad. You do a great job. What are your plans for the holidays?"

He took a deep breath, held it for a moment, and said, "I'm going home."

"Home to Brazil?"

He smiled, adjusting his glasses. "Yes, Brazil. I haven't seen my mother in twelve years."

"But if you go you can't come back, can you?"

"No. I have no visa."

Roman's vacation visa had expired a few months after he first got to the United States over twelve years ago. He managed to stay with the help of the woman he worked for. If he left and went back to Brazil he could not return to the United States. Once in a while he'd mentioned his wish to go home, to see his mother and his friends, but he worried about having HIV there, getting care. He worried about being able to find work. Brazil, however, unlike many other countries, had made a commitment to caring for patients with HIV in the early 1990s. All patients had access to medications. Brazil's forward-thinking and aggressive treatment programs kept its infection rates very low and made it a leader among countries having large indigent populations. In contrast, the president of South Africa, in the early 1990s, had declared that the AIDS epidemic simply did not exist. His government did not support HIV education or prevention and treatment programs, with the result that in many poor communities of South Africa the HIV infection rates approached 30 percent by the end of the decade.

I didn't worry that Roman was returning to Brazil; I felt confident that he'd get excellent care and be able to continue all his medications. If anything, he might find less stigma there as well, given Brazil's open acknowledgment of the epidemic.

"Roman, I'm really glad for you. And I'm glad for your mother. She'll be happy to see you, I'd imagine."

Roman laughed and the blue of his eyes was not obscured by any purple spot or scar, a far different image from what had been the case three years ago. Before he left he gave me a hug. I wished him luck and told him that we'd miss him. Roman had done all the hard work just by taking his medicine. I couldn't hope to fix what was broken for so many of my patients. I cheered when the virus became undetectable, but prescriptions couldn't heal a broken home or an abusive childhood or ten years in jail for drug possession. Roman had a healthy life and I didn't have many patients like him.

Olive had been taken down from CSS in a wheelchair to get a chest X-ray and from there would be going directly to a hospital room. I would be seeing her and Etta and a couple of other patients in the hospital shortly. Before I went to see my inpatients, Stewart was my last clinic appointment of the morning. He came into the office carrying a cane in his left hand. He didn't touch the ground with it and he didn't limp.

"Stewart, why are you carrying the cane?"

"Oh." He glanced at it as if surprised to see it there in his hand. "Oh, this? I have it because sometimes my leg feels weak. I have some neuropathy, Dr. Ball, they told me I have some neuropathy so I have the cane."

"Who's they?"

"Who?"

"You said they told you that you have neuropathy. Who's they?"

"Oh. My therapist at the massage center. I go there every week. My massage therapist gave me the cane." Stewart had gotten himself plugged in to a slew of support organizations. He had yoga and massage, meal deliveries, lunches at this or that community-based organization, and all kinds of meetings for people with HIV. In an odd way HIV had become a kind of focal point for Stewart's daily life. Whereas some patients wanted as few reminders of HIV as possible, for others HIV kept them alive. Stewart had filled his life with HIV-related services. I couldn't imagine what kind of person he'd be, or how he'd spend his time, if he didn't have this entire network to keep him occupied.

"OK," I said. "It just looks as if you aren't actually using it. Do you carry it just in case?"

"Yeah. Just in case."

"And how are you feeling otherwise, Stewart? Are things going OK?"

His forehead took on its characteristic furrow as his eyebrows poked up to his hairline. "Dr. Ball, this thing with my sugar has me very worried. I haven't been eating desserts or drinking soda, I don't understand how I could have high sugar. Why do you think this is happening?"

Stewart's blood sugar measurements revealed the development of diabetes and I'd gotten the nurses to teach him how to check his sugar with a finger prick and a glucose monitor. Despite his rigid adherence to his HIV medications, he wanted to ignore this new development in his health. He resisted the teaching, didn't check his glucose as often as I would have liked, and he did not want to consider the idea that he might be diabetic.

"Stewart, it's good that you're watching what you eat. Diet's important in diabetes—"

"Are you saying I have diabetes? Dr. Ball, I don't think I have diabetes."

"Well, Stewart, your sugars are in a range where we'd say that you do. Even with watching your diet your sugars have been over one fifty. I'm going to make you an appointment to see the endocrinologist. You have what we call type two or adult-onset diabetes. Usually we can manage it with oral medication. I'm going to send you to see Miranda, too. Your diet is important and a diabetic diet is more than just watching out for sweets and desserts. She'll tell you all about it."

The look on Stewart's face while I talked was as if he were watching someone being dismembered. He ran a trembling hand through his thin, stringy hair and shook his head. "This is very upsetting to me, Dr. Ball. I just don't understand how I could be diabetic. I haven't had dessert in two weeks. Could it be from the Coumadin? Could the Coumadin be giving me diabetes?"

"No, it's not the Coumadin. But your HIV may have something to do with it. There have been increasing cases of diabetes in patients with HIV, particularly patients on protease inhibitors."

"The indinavir could be causing this?"

"It's not clear. Not yet, anyway. And right now no one is suggesting that people stop taking their HIV medication. We can treat the high sugar. And you need to keep your viral load under control."

"It's under control, isn't it?" Stewart again looked agitated and his eyebrows seemed to have their own agenda. "I haven't missed any doses. I take the indinavir faithfully."

"Yes, your viral load is fine. You do a great job taking your medicine. I don't want you to stop. As I say, you might need to add a new medication for the sugar, but we aren't telling people to stop their HIV medications."

"What new medicine? Does it have side effects?"

I silently groaned, thinking, uh-oh, what have I just started? "There are several things to choose from so I'm going to let the specialist be the one to suggest what you should take. Given your history and the fairly mild elevations of your sugar, I'd like to get their input."

Stewart sat shaking his head. "Oh, this is terrible." He looked back up at me almost beseechingly.

"Stewart," I said, "try to settle down. This isn't a catastrophe. It's a disease that we can treat and take care of. You're someone who does a fantastic job taking your medicine. Look at your viral load; you've done beautifully. You take the Coumadin and the blood pressure medicine. It's another pill, yes, it's another condition to have to be aware of, but you keep your appointments and take care of yourself. It's going to be fine. You can't ignore it or pretend it isn't happening, but it's going to be fine."

He nodded hesitantly as I spoke. His anxiety and relentless worrying could be hard to take but his neurosis provoked a vigilant approach to taking medications. Although his T cells had not gone up very much on his HIV regimen, his virus never rose to detectable levels.

I examined Stewart and continued to try sounding optimistic, even cajoling, to get that furrow in his brow to relax a bit. He left my office heading down the hall to see Zoe Prin. She had him on a low dose of an antianxiety medication. Despite his initial aversion to new or different medications, once he was on something he took it faithfully. He would have taken much more of the antianxiety medication but Zoe and I agreed that probably all the Valium in the world would not make Stewart any less anxious. I joked that we couldn't give it all to Stewart when we might and did need some of it ourselves.

My phone rang as I completed my chart notes from the morning patients. "Dr. Ball? It's Terry. Ms. B. just passed away."

"Oh, wow." I said it softly, completely floored.

"The nurse had just been in the room—they'd been able to move her to a private room—and said she seemed more somnolent. Her blood pressure was a little bit lower but not alarming. Still, when she went back in, the patient had no pulse. I've called her mother, who's coming now."

"You spoke to her mother already?"

"I called her at her work number."

"Oh, wow. This is a sad story. How was she?"

"She seemed OK. Maybe a little businesslike. She was at work, but she thanked me and said she'd come right away."

"So can you leave Etta where she is for now? Until her mother gets here?"

"Yeah, the nurses are fine for now. They like the mother and they'll wait for her to come."

"Thanks for letting me know, Terry. I'll be there shortly, too."

"Dr. Ball, I saw your other patient, Ms. G.?"

I tried to focus. Terry was also taking care of Olive. Etta was dead but Olive was sick and I needed to collect my thoughts for her. "Yes, good. Did you get her ABG?"

"It's cooking and should be back any minute. My resident, though, wanted to get a MICU consult for her just in case."

"That's fine. A good idea. Go ahead and start her on pentamidine and depending on the ABG we can see if she needs steroids and possibly a bed in the ICU. Cover her also for atypicals, given her recent trip. Will pulmonary see her?"

"The fellow's with her now."

"Great. Thank you, Terry, I appreciate it."

"Ms. G. has a lot of charts." As an intern, Terry would have called for the old charts for her new inpatient. The electronic medical record in the hospital was relatively new and most patients' old charts had not been scanned into the computer. Probably two or three fat charts attesting to Olive's very long history had been brought to the floor for the resident and intern to look at. The poor intern no doubt wondered where she'd possibly get the time to go through all that material.

"Oh, Olive has a lot of charts. She does indeed. Don't get too crazed about it, though. Olive's a very interesting patient but her current problem is hopefully fairly straightforward. She's sick, so keep a close eye on her. I'll be seeing her there soon as well."

"OK, Dr. Ball, thanks."

I hung up the phone and looked out the window behind my desk. How many times had I done that in these last eight years? Every day, at some point in the day, I looked at the river, at the airport in the distance, at the cars down on York Avenue. When it rained I watched as the drops ran down the glass; the headlights of the cars made the wet street far below look shiny. A few times a peregrine falcon stopped on the ledge outside my window. Its legs are bright yellow, its beak extremely pointed. We watched each other closely, the wind ruffling the bird's feathers as it turned its head from side to side. Today I looked out at another soggy December sky, the streets dark and gloomy. They said it might snow later tonight. I did not want to think about Etta being dead. I turned back to my computer and finished my notes. Then I put on my white coat and took the elevator to the inpatient floor.

Much later that night I sat in my living room in the dark as the boys slept. Shari and I had had a late dinner and she'd gone to bed, anticipating an early start in the labor room in the morning. I sat on our couch and heard the occasional car on Broadway. The rain continued. Images of the last hours ran through my head like a series of video clips. Olive wearing a nasal oxygen tube, resting quietly in her bed, the single light behind her pillow flickering through the clear plastic of the three IV bags hanging from a pole next to her. My relief that she didn't need to go to the ICU, but what could be in store for her if I couldn't get her to take her medication?

Another image in the video clips was of the new patient, Davidson. Just after leaving my office on my way to see the inpatients, I'd been called to see a consult for a new patient with HIV. A gay man in his forties, Davidson had an enormous KS lesion growing in the back of his mouth, palpable under his chin and extending down his neck. He acknowledged losing eighty pounds, claiming he'd been on a diet. Testing positive for HIV in 1993, he hadn't gone back to the doctor, and despite his almost complete inability to swallow, he behaved as if the growth in his mouth belonged to someone else. I found myself more than surprised that a person could ignore his health so dramatically. I didn't tell him that just a few weeks ago another patient of mine had died from untreated KS. I didn't tell this patient about Sabir, dying at home with his mother and sisters at his side, praying for him and crying. I felt angry at this Davidson patient. What kind of person neglects himself in such a thoroughly destructive way?

But the video clip that played over and over in my mind was the one where I got to Etta's floor and walked past the nurses' station toward her room. Mrs. B. is coming toward me. She is a short, stocky woman, built like Etta before Etta lost so much weight. She wears an unbuttoned khaki overcoat and she carries a maroon scarf in her hands. Mrs. B with short, styled gray hair that once was dyed brown, and wire-rimmed glasses. She looks up and sees me coming toward her. All the thoughts crashing through my head. What can I say to this woman whose daughter is now gone forever? Who will take care of the children? Joey climbing into the cupboard beneath the sink. Little Etta. Never to know the feisty, exasperating character of her mother. I'm a mother and cannot begin to know what this mother is feeling. I'm a doctor and there has been so much loss. Losing Etta feels like losing everyone all at once. I reach out to hug Mrs. B. and she hugs me back. Missing a daughter, missing a mother, we stand there weeping. In my living room I am crying again. For Etta and her mother. For my mother. For Sabir and Peaches and Brandon's patient who didn't make it home to Africa. For Bella and Cecil, Marta and Luz and their children. I think of Timothy who would have been my friend.

There are not many nights like this. I put my head back against the couch and look out at the city streetlights casting long shadows on the ceiling. All the faces and memories flow past and over me; I am changed, I am the same. I feel thankful. To Etta and Peaches, Roman and Stewart, and so many others over these years. All of my patients. All I've learned, all I've experienced. I wish some things had worked out differently, but I can resolve only to listen and keep learning. So much I've seen and so much more still to see. In this moment I am overwhelmed with a feeling of gratefulness. A sense that I've been privileged. It's late and I'm tired. I'll go check on Olive in the morning before I see my first patients in the office. I get up and make my way through the dark apartment to kiss the boys and go to bed.

# Epilogue

It is ten years later and I am on call for the weekend. It's nearly noon and I'm headed home, walking west through Central Park, having seen all the inpatients on my list who needed to be seen. I'm not on call on the weekend very much these days. Stan and I have been around the longest and I guess it's a perk of being more senior. My younger colleagues spread out the coverage among them. But aside from that, the weekends are not what they used to be. It's not four or six in the evening, for one thing. And I saw ten patients, not thirty. There are other patients in the hospital with HIV but they don't require a visit from me on Saturday.

Central Park is so vibrant in early May. The apple and redbud trees are in bloom and the grass is looking shimmery and lush. Birds chase one another and near the castle the turtles poke their heads out of the dark pond. I saw a snowy egret last week. It always reminds me of my mother to see that bright white narrow bird outlined against the reeds, stepping around soundlessly in the shallow water.

One of the patients this morning brought back such a strong reminder of what AIDS can do, of what AIDS did to so many, many people. She could not have been more than thirty-five but had the grayish skin and dry hair of an old woman. She held a pencil poised over her menu choices for the hospital lunch and she looked at me with fierce, determined eyes.

"I done cooked all day yesterday and them people came and ate every last bite." She looked furtively to her left. "Ain't no more shrimps. Ain't no more crabs. They ain't nothin'." She looked to her right. The nurse's aide sitting next to her looked at me and rolled her eyes. I knew from my sign-out sheet that the woman had been admitted last week after the family found they could not care for her. She'd had HIV for ten years and never taken medication for more than a day or two. She probably weighed about eighty pounds and her brain scan showed the classic shrinking of advanced AIDS. She talked constantly of "going home tomorrow." She hadn't recognized her children when they came to visit.

Another patient smiled bravely at me when I walked into her room. She then leaned over and gagged into the basin at her side. She had metastatic breast cancer and unremitting nausea from her treatment. Even in her dark skin the circles around her eyes looked black. HIV was a minor consideration for this woman. For some reason, out of the blue I thought of Luz, my patient from long ago who died of hepatitis C. Everyone was afraid of her because she had HIV. But it was something else entirely that killed her. She never told her family, fearing their rejection. I wondered if the woman in front of me had told her family about her HIV. Her morphine doses were being increased almost daily to keep her comfortable and she will probably die within a few months from her cancer. Increasingly, HIV is not the cause of death for our patients.

I stop at the Great Lawn and watch four boys playing soccer together, expertly kicking the ball to one another, bouncing it off their knees or their ankles before sending it to the next one. Nearby two women are lying on the grass with their shoes off, chatting. All around me people play catch, sit in the sun, take pictures of one another.

I look back at the boys playing soccer and think of Nathan and Jason, their parents, Bella and Cecil, long dead from AIDS. Jason, the younger brother, is now my colleague's patient. He spent a lot of his teenage years rebelling against everything and everyone. A few months ago his older brother, Nathan, called Dr. Berry, totally out of the blue. She no longer works at CSS but he'd tracked her down and asked her for help to get Jason back into care. Jason was in the hospital for a while, his HIV highly resistant from his stopping and starting various medications over the years. I'd seen him one day in the hospital. He had no idea who I was and seemed uninterested when I told him that I'd taken care of his parents in the past. Perhaps he still blames them; I don't know. My colleague put together a regimen for Jason with some new drugs and now he's doing well. Maybe someday I will know him better and be able to tell him how much his parents loved him.

Stewart was in the hospital last week. He had a urinary tract infection that made his diabetes go wild and he developed severe dehydration that nearly ruined his kidneys. For a day or two I really worried about him, but with antibiotics and fluids he recovered beautifully. His viral load has been undetectable now for ten years. He takes the same protease inhibitor that I first prescribed for him, refusing to take anything else even though now I could give him fewer pills that he'd have to take only once a day. I tried a few times to get him to consider something simpler, but after endless questions and watching those worried eyebrows I stopped suggesting. We don't say "Hit early, hit hard" anymore. With Stewart I say, "It's not broken, don't fix it." This makes him laugh.

The frail, demented woman I saw today reminded me a bit of Sabitha, so small and so hard to reach. Sabitha died about five years after she left the nursing home. She'd taken her medications for a few months and then stopped. Her disease staggered along, progressing in increments and never really getting much better. Her daughter Monica and one of the boys became parents before they were in their twenties. Sabitha enjoyed seeing the babies but she didn't stay around long enough to see very much of them.

We now talk about HIV being a chronic disease. In other parts of the world AIDS continues to kill millions of people every year, but in the United States more and more people are living with HIV because they're taking their medication and are doing fine. Patients who have HIV often die from another cause; cancer, say, or heart disease. Still, more than fifteen thousand die from HIV-related illness every year. Many of these deaths occur in people who aren't taking their medication, or who aren't taking it correctly.

I recently saw Olive in the office. Ten years ago I would not have thought it possible that she'd be alive a decade later, given her persistently elevated viral loads and her resistance to more and more medications. Sometime after her hospitalization for PCP, though, something seemed to click for her. Her numbers started improving and she was apparently taking her medications without missing any doses. Her regimen is not easy; she takes a lot of pills. But she's been doing well. She also stopped coming into my office with new, weird complaints. She goes on a cruise every so often and I admire the pictures when she gets back.

I don't miss those bad old days of HIV care. Even just the few patients I've seen today remind me of the sad, hollow feeling of watching so many young people dying from an illness we could not treat. But in the 1980s and early 1990s it had been like trekking on another planet, exploring unknown territory where few wanted to go. Our precious camaraderie bonded us together; bonded us, too, with our patients, as we tried to help and protect them. Maybe it's a bit like the metaphor of the battlefield, where we shared a sense of being alive, of doing something brave and important. Today our care for our patients can become routine. We spend a lot of time talking about taking pills and stopping smoking. The feeling of serving on a unique and noble battlefront has diminished. I recognize that we have good medications, effective treatment for HIV, but there is much in my patients' lives that goes untreated. For so many, AIDS is one symptom in a life of limited opportunities, unmet needs, and inequities. Still, it gets no less hard to see patients dying from this disease.

The park is so beautiful today. My beeper goes off; it's a patient requesting that I call in a refill of his medications to his pharmacy. As I dial I look up and see the egret lifting off from the edge of the pond, its heavy white wings beating at the air and long black legs trailing behind. It circles and rises, now looking like a handkerchief flapping and waving into the sky.

In rounds after clinic the other day we were slowly going through the long list of patients, this one doing well, that one needing detox, another asking for help with her bills. Carl is a physician who works with us now. He's a superb doctor with a very dry wit. He barely cracked a smile as he presented his patient, a man with the same name as a famous deceased politician, who believes that he is the love child of that politician and his lover, an iconic actress. Carl's mouth twitched up slightly as he concluded by saying that the patient's HIV is under good control on medication.

Further along in rounds we heard about the man who wears sunglasses and is never without his Seeing Eye dog, but who is not blind. Around the table there were puzzled looks and chuckles of disbelief.

Not for the first time, and I'm sure not for the last, I thought, every day at my job something happens that I could not have imagined.

"Fuckin' A," said Stan, shaking his head and leaning back in his chair.

We move on to the next patient.